Pain Management

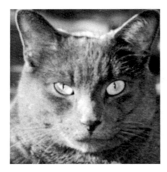

for the Small Animal Practitioner
Second Edition

by

William J. Tranquilli,
DVM, MS, Diplomate, ACVA

Kurt A. Grimm,
DVM, MS, PhD, Diplomate, ACVA, ACVCP

Leigh A. Lamont,
DVM, MS, Diplomate, ACVA

T0132735

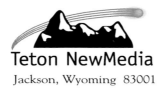

Teton NewMedia
Jackson, Wyoming 83001

Executive Editor: Carroll C. Cann
Development Editor: Susan L. Hunsberger
Editor: Cynthia J. Roantree
Design: Anita Sykes
Layout: 5640 Design – www.fiftysixforty.com

Made Easy Series Editors:
Larry P. Tilley, DVM, Diplomate ACVIM (Internal Medicine)
Francis W.K. Smith Jr., DVM, Diplomate ACVIM (Cardiology and Internal Medicine)

Teton NewMedia
P.O. Box 4833
4125 South Hwy 89
Jackson, WY 83001

1-888-770-3165
www.tetonewmedia.com
www.veterinarywire.com

Illustrations by Kerry Helms

PRINTED IN THE UNITED STATES OF AMERICA

Print number 5 4 3

         Library of Congress Cataloging-in-Publication Data
Tranquilli, William J.
      Pain Management for the small animal practitioner / by William J. Tranquilli, Kurt A. Grimm, Leigh A. Lamont. --2nd ed.
         p. ; cm. -- (Made Easy Series)
      Includes bibliographical references and index.
      ISBN 1-59161-024-9
      1. Dogs--Diseases--Treatment. 2. Cats--Diseases--Treatment. 3. Pain in animals. I. Grimm,Kurt A. II. Lamont, Leigh A. III. Title IV. Made easy series (Jackson, Wyo.)
      [DNLM: 1. Analgesia--veterinary--Handbooks. 2. Pain--veterinary--Handbooks. 3. Analgesics--therapeutic use--Handbooks. 4. Cats--Handbooks. 5. Dogs--Handbooks. SF 910.P34 T772p 2004]
      SF991.T75 2004
      636.7'0896'0472--dc22

                                                                    2004048006

Dedication

The second edition of this book continues to be dedicated to the small animal practitioner working to advance veterinary pain management and to all of our beloved pets who deserve compassionate care.

William J. Tranquilli
Kurt A. Grimm
Leigh A. Lamont

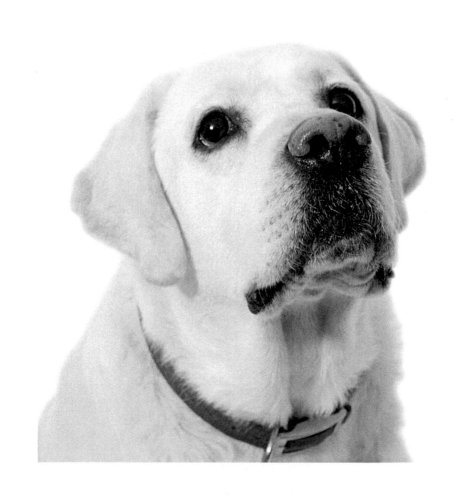

Preface

This past decade has seen pain management emerge as a key issue in veterinary medicine. Since the publication of the first edition of this handbook in 2000 our understanding of the processes both mediating and alleviating pain have continued to evolve. Although we continue to recognize that our knowledge of animal pain and its treatment is incomplete, efforts to improve the quality of animal care through the alleviation of pain has proven beneficial to our patients and is greatly appreciated by pet owners. It is our hope that the updated information contained in the second edition of this handbook will further guide the practitioner in the everyday management of patient pain and discomfort.

The authors wish to express their gratitude to the anesthesiology faculty and staff of the University of Illinois' College of Veterinary Medicine Teaching Hospital and to all those veterinarians committed to advancing the field of veterinary pain management.

Table of Contents

Section 1 Pain Terminology, Physiology, Recognition, and Clinical Strategies for Management

Section 2 Analgesic Drugs

Section 3 Analgesic Techniques

Section 4 Pain Management for Specific
Conditions and Procedures

Section 5 Managing Chronic Pain
in Dogs and Cats

Section 6 Implementing a Pain Management
Program in Clinical Practice

Appendix

Index

Recommended Readings

Introduction

The goals of this book

are to provide the veterinary practitioner with a description of
common pain syndromes, review the drugs and techniques used to
treat pain, and suggest ways to manage pain arising from a variety
of surgical procedures, trauma, and diseases. By applying the
concepts and techniques presented in this book, veterinarians will
be better able to communicate the importance of pain recognition and
management to the pet owner while providing better analgesic therapy
and compassionate care to their patients.

Some Helpful Hints

Throughout the text you will find the following symbols
to help you focus on what is really important.

✓ This is a routine feature of the subject being discussed.
We've tried to narrow it down, honest.

♥ This is a salient feature. If you remember anything about
this particular subject, this is it.

🖤 Something serious, possibly life-threatening, will happen
if you don't remember this. For example, a fatal drug
interaction may occur when an NSAID and a steroid are
co-administered.

⊙ A CD is available as an accompaniment to this printed
volume. The CD-ROM allows you to search and retrieve
the full text, figures, and tables of the book, plus 11 videos
demonstrating Analgesic Techniques. To purchase this
CD-ROM, please call 877-306-9793.

Section 1

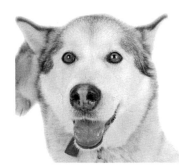

Pain Terminology, Physiology, Recognition, and Clinical Strategies for Management

Pain Terminology

The International Association for the Study of Pain (IASP) has defined pain as an unpleasant sensory or emotional experience associated with actual or potential tissue damage, or described in terms of such damage.

Some definitions commonly used to characterize pain, its treatment, and its consequences are:

Allodynia – Pain produced by non-noxious stimuli.

Analgesia – Absence of pain sensation.

Distress – Physical and emotional display of physical or mental strain or stress.

Hyperesthesia – Increased sensitivity to non-noxious stimuli.

Hyperalgesia – Increased pain response to a noxious stimulus either at the site of injury (primary) or in surrounding undamaged tissue (secondary).

Hypoalgesia – Reduced pain sensation.

Stress – Physical or mental discomfort.

Suffering – Endurance of physical or mental strain or stress.

✓ Classifications of pain are based upon anatomic origin or physiologic significance:

Physiologic (Nociceptive) pain is produced by stimulation of nociceptors innervated by high-threshold A-delta and unmyelinated C fibers. The sensation of pain protects the body by warning of contact with tissue-damaging stimuli (teaching pain).

Pathologic (Clinical) pain is caused by the ongoing activation of nociceptors due to peripheral tissue injury or injury to the nervous system. Both peripheral and neuropathic pain can produce alterations in nervous system function resulting in allodynia, hyperalgesia, and central and peripheral sensitization.

Peripheral pain is either visceral (thoracic and abdominal viscera) or somatic (joints, muscles, or periosteum). Visceral pain is poorly localized and is frequently described as cramping or gnawing. Visceral pain may also be referred to cutaneous sites far from the site of injury. Somatic pain is easily localized, and is often described as acute, aching, stabbing, or throbbing. Somatic pain includes cutaneous pain after an operation. Somatic pain can be further classified as superficial (skin) or deep (joints, muscle, periosteum) in origin.

Neuropathic pain can result from trauma, inflammation or sensitization of peripheral nerves or spinal cord. Neuropathic pain is described as burning, lancinating, and intermittent, and is often poorly responsive to treatment.

Idiopathic pain persists in the absence of an identifiable organic substrate. Idiopathic pain is often excessive and associated with emotional stress or behavioral abnormalities.

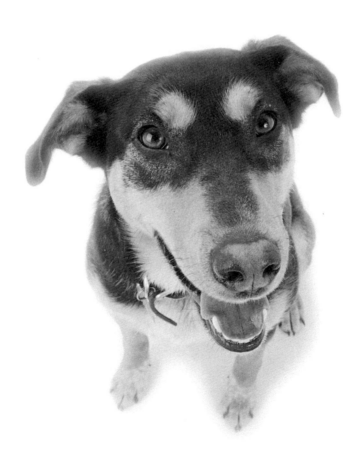

Physiology of Pain
The Sensory
Nervous System and Pain

✓ Simplistically, nociceptive pathways can be considered as a three neuron-chain, with the first order neuron originating in the periphery and projecting to the spinal cord, the second order neuron ascending the spinal cord, and the third order neuron projecting into the cerebral cortex and other supraspinal structures (Figure 1-1). On a more complex level, the pathway involves a network of branches and communications with other sensory neurons and descending inhibitory neurons from the midbrain which modulate afferent transmission of painful stimuli. The first process of pain recognition involves encoding mechanical, chemical, or thermal energy into electrical impulses by specialized nerve endings termed nociceptors. These receptors exist as free nerve endings of primary afferent neurons and function by signaling actual or potential tissue injury. These signals are transmitted by small diameter, myelinated A-delta axons that conduct impulses very rapidly producing what is often referred to as "first pain." Transmission in smaller, unmyelinated C-fibers is much slower, referred to as "second pain" and reinforces the immediate response produced by A-delta fibers. Both A-delta and C-fibers are found throughout the skin, peritoneum, pleura, periosteum, subchondral bone, joint capsules, blood vessels, muscles, tendons, fascia, and viscera. Cell bodies of both types of afferent fibers are contained in the dorsal root ganglia and extend axons to synapse with dorsal horn neurons within the gray matter of the spinal cord. It is in the dorsal horn that initial integration and modulation of nociceptive input occurs. Primary afferents form direct or indirect connections with one of three populations of dorsal horn neurons: (1) interneurons that may be either excitatory or inhibitory; (2) propriospinal neurons involved in segmented reflex activity; and (3) projection neurons that extend to supraspinal centers such as the midbrain and cortex. These projection neurons are divided into several ascending tracts, including the spinothalamic tract, the spinomesencephalic tract, and the spinocervical tract. These neurons synapse with third order neurons located in portions of the medulla, pons, midbrain, thalamus and hypothalamus, and cerebral cortex where pain is ultimately perceived. Painful afferent stimuli are subject to an array of diverse inhibitory influences by the descending modulatory system. Inhibition occurs within cortical and thalamic structures, midbrain, rostral medulla and brainstem, and the spinal cord dorsal horn. In summary, pain ascends via a three-neuron chain with dual excitatory and inhibitory input at each level.

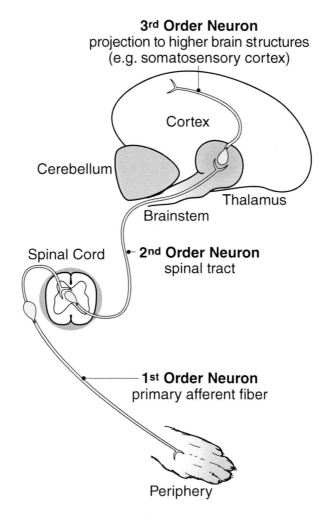

3rd Order Neuron
projection to higher brain structures
(e.g. somatosensory cortex)

Cortex

Cerebellum

Thalamus

Brainstem

Spinal Cord

2nd Order Neuron
spinal tract

1st Order Neuron
primary afferent fiber

Periphery

Figure 1-1
A simplified representation of the afferent pain pathway

Nociception

✓ Nociception is the transduction, conduction, and central nervous system processing of signals generated by the stimulation of nociceptors (Figure 1-2). It is the physiologic process that, when carried to completion, results in the conscious perception of pain. Because the anatomic structures and neurophysiologic mechanisms leading to the perception of pain (nociception) are remarkably similar in human beings and animals, it is reasonable to assume that a stimulus that is painful to people, is damaging or potentially damaging to tissues, and induces escape and behavioral responses in an animal, must be considered painful to that animal. Nociception consists of three distinct physiologic processes that are subject to pharmacologic modulation.

Transduction is the translation of physical energy (noxious stimuli) into electrical activity at the peripheral nociceptor. These receptors are considered mechanosensitive, thermosensitive, and chemosensitive.

Transmission is the propagation of nerve impulses through the nervous system. Afferent sensory fibers consist of myelinated A-delta fibers which conduct fast pain, and nonmyelinated C fibers which conduct slower dull pain.

Modulation occurs through the endogenous descending analgesic systems, which modify nociceptive transmission. These endogenous systems (opioid, serotonergic, and noradrenergic) modulate nociception through the inhibition of stimuli processing within spinal dorsal horn cells.

Perception, although not considered a part of the nociceptive process, results from successful transduction, transmission, modulation, and integration of thalamocortical, reticular, and limbic function to produce the final conscious subjective and emotional experience of pain. Nociceptive input is modulated at every level of the sensory pathway, from the periphery to the cerebral cortex where perception occurs.

Although the behavior of nonprimate mammals implies that they experience "feelings" (emotional or moral sensitivity) from the body in the same way as humans, neuroanatomical evidence indicates otherwise as the phylogenetically new pathways conveying homeostatic afferent activity directly to the thalamocortical levels in primates is either rudimentary or absent in nonprimates. Said in another way, although the perception of pain occurs the "feelings" it engenders in our pets is possibly different from humans. This concept continues to be debated among neuroscientists and veterinarians.

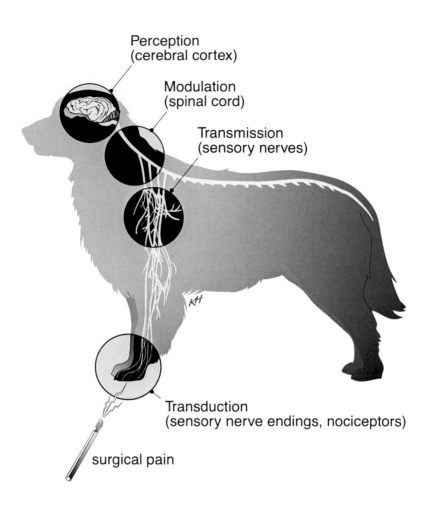

Perception
(cerebral cortex)

Modulation
(spinal cord)

Transmission
(sensory nerves)

Transduction
(sensory nerve endings, nociceptors)

surgical pain

Figure 1-2
Physiologic processes of pain recognition

Consequences of Pain

When pain becomes pathologic in nature, a variety of consequences may ensue including: increased risk of infection, delayed wound healing, reduced food and water intake, immobilization, altered sleep patterns, and change from normal behavior patterns. Many of these changes prolong convalescence and predispose the patient to an adverse outcome.

Pain Recognition

✓ Physiologic signs of acute pain include increased blood pressure, heart rate, and peripheral vasoconstriction that manifests itself as blanched mucus membranes. Respiratory rate often increases and muscle splinting may occur if pain is localized within the thorax.

✓ A stress leukogram is often evident and catabolic processes predominate.

♥ Responses to pain vary among species, but a variety of behaviors and signs are consistent with ongoing painful conditions. Alterations in normal vocalization patterns and attention-seeking behaviors are common. Dogs often whine or whimper while cats groom, growl, or purr. Dogs can become either timid or aggressive toward human interactive behavior. Cats often try to hide when in pain. Facial expressions and body posture can be quite revealing as dogs may have a fixed stare and arching posture whereas cats may squint their eyes and refuse to move. Dogs and cats both demonstrate guarding behaviors of injured or painful tissues by biting or scratching when palpated and often lick, chew, or paw at the site of pain. Some dogs become restless while cats often refuse to interact or change body positions.

✓ Pain can reduce appetite and food intake, alter voiding behaviors, and reduce grooming behaviors so that the patient appears disheveled.

✓ Given the complexity of pain perception, behavioral signs of pain are unique for each animal and may be best identified by the animal's owner. It is unlikely that a single reliable objective measure of pain exists, and few correlations between subjective and objective measures of pain severity have been documented.

✓ When there is a likelihood of experiencing postoperative pain, analgesics should be used regardless of an animal's outward behavior. Generally the benefits of pain management outweigh the risks associated with analgesic drug administration.

Pain Assessment

✓ The practitioner should become familiar with the patient's normal and/or presenting physiologic values and behaviors by assessing these parameters at admission.

✓ A thorough pain assessment should include both a non-interactive evaluation carried out from a distance, and a interactive evaluation that encourages a response from the patient.

✓ A series of assessments should be made and recorded in the medical record at appropriate intervals to document changes in pain status and response to therapy. It is recommended that serial pain assessments be made by the same observer, if possible, to reduce inter-observer differences.

✓ Several simple pain assessment tools have been used clinically to evaluate pain and distress in veterinary patients. These include the visual analog scale (VAS) and the numerical rating scale (NRS).

✓ The VAS is comprised of a line of a standard length, usually 10 cm, upon which a mark is made to indicate the observer's impression of the intensity of pain the patient is experiencing. The distance from the end to the mark is measured and recorded as the pain score. It is important for all users to understand the meaning of the end point of the line (e.g., worst pain imaginable or worst pain possible for a particular condition). Inter-observer variation will occur, but can be minimized by training users. This tool can be used rapidly and in many different clinical situations.

✓ The NRS is similar to the VAS in that it is a line of standard length; however, the line is divided at regular intervals by numbers that usually range from 0 to 10. Some scales add descriptions of the expected behaviors at points on the line to aid in assessment. The NRS is usually more repeatable when used by multiple observers.

Strategies for Pain Management

Preemptive Analgesia

✓ Preemptive analgesia refers to the application of analgesic techniques before the patient is exposed to noxious stimuli (e.g., surgical trespass). This decreases the intensity and duration of post-procedure pain and minimizes the likelihood of a chronic pain state being established. Examples of preemptive analgesic techniques include the use of anesthetic premedication such as opioids, alpha$_2$ agonists, and NSAIDs, or the presurgical epidural administration of local anesthetics or opioids. Remember that preemptive analgesia cannot eliminate postoperative pain, but can help prevent peripheral and central nervous system sensitization during the surgical procedure. This concept has gained acceptance as an effective method to improve perianesthetic pain management.

Multimodal Analgesia

✓ Balanced, or multimodal, analgesia is achieved by the simultaneous administration of two or more analgesic drug classes or techniques. Since various classes of drugs such as NSAIDs, opioids, alpha$_2$ agonists, and local anesthetics have additive or synergistic analgesic effects when co administered, dosages can typically be reduced. The rationale behind multimodal analgesia arises from the fact that inhibition of nociception can be achieved at different points along the afferent pain pathway through distinct mechanisms. For example, transduction can be inhibited by NSAIDs, transmission obtunded by peripheral nerve block with a local anesthetic, and modulation enhanced by the co-administration of opioids and alpha$_2$ agonists (Figure 1-3). This is analogous to using several antineoplastic agents in the same patient to inhibit tumor cell metabolism and replication through different mechanisms. When used preemptively, balanced analgesia helps to (1) prevent or inhibit surgery-induced peripheral nociceptor sensitization (inflammation) and neuroplastic changes within the spinal cord (wind up); (2) prevent development of tachyphylaxis (i.e., loss of efficacy); (3) suppress the neuroendocrine stress response to pain and injury; and (4) shorten convalescence through improved tissue healing (decreased catabolic process), maintenance of immune responses (decreased infection), and improved patient mobility. Multimodal analgesic strategies are equally applicable in managing acute or chronic refractory pain syndromes.

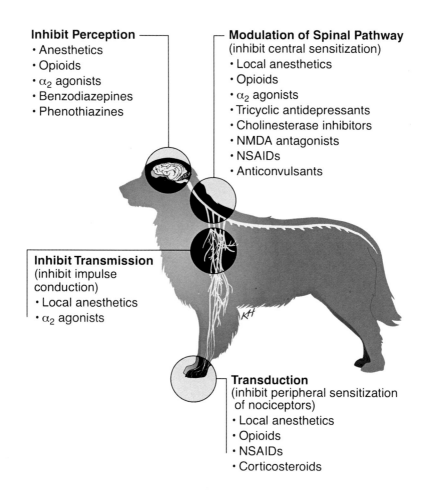

Inhibit Perception
• Anesthetics
• Opioids
• α_2 agonists
• Benzodiazepines
• Phenothiazines

Modulation of Spinal Pathway
(inhibit central sensitization)
• Local anesthetics
• Opioids
• α_2 agonists
• Tricyclic antidepressants
• Cholinesterase inhibitors
• NMDA antagonists
• NSAIDs
• Anticonvulsants

Inhibit Transmission
(inhibit impulse conduction)
• Local anesthetics
• α_2 agonists

Transduction
(inhibit peripheral sensitization of nociceptors)
• Local anesthetics
• Opioids
• NSAIDs
• Corticosteroids

Figure 1-3
Pharmacologic intervention of pain processing

Placebo Effect

✓ The term placebo literally translates to "I shall please." All proposed mechanisms for the placebo effect suggest an interaction of brain states and somatic health processes (Table 1-1).

Table 1-1 Some Proposed Mechanisms for the Placebo Effect in Animals
Human Contact – Visual and tactile contact from a human can cause changes in the subject's physiologic state, response to painful stimuli, and productivity.
Classical Conditioning – Pavlov first demonstrated classical conditioning with morphine in dogs. Classical conditioning usually requires repeated exposures to the conditioned stimulus and therefore may be a factor in chronic pain treatment.
Endogenous opioids – This mechanism may explain analgesic placebo responses, but not physiologic responses such as immune modulation or tissue healing.

✓ When objective and subjective pain assessment scores improve with the administration of a placebo, interpretation of the effectiveness of analgesic treatment is difficult.

✓ Expectancy (a probable mechanism of the placebo effect in humans) requires the ability of the patient to comprehend and anticipate a response to a treatment (e.g., faith or hope). The existence of expectancy in animals is questionable. However, expectancy may lead to observer bias when assessing response to treatment.

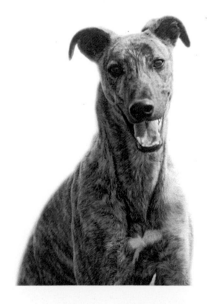

Section 2

Analgesic Drugs

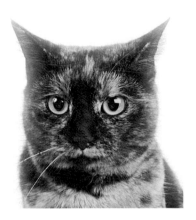

Opioids

Mechanisms of Action

✓ Opioids act primarily at pre- and postsynaptic receptors present in the peripheral and central nervous systems. All opioids have a similar mode of action, though activity at various receptor subtypes varies. Currently three opioid receptors have been cloned, OP1 (δ), OP2 (κ), OP3 (μ) that are known to mediate analgesia. Activation of opioid receptors by either an exogenous opioid agonist or endogenous ligand inhibits the presynaptic release of excitatory neurotransmitters from nerve terminals in the dorsal horn of the spinal cord (See Figure 5-1). Inhibition occurs as the result of hyperpolarization mediated by increased potassium conductance and/or calcium channel inactivation. Opioids do not appear to impair conduction of stimuli along afferent sensory nerves. (See Table 2-1 for dosages and indications of commonly used opioids in veterinary medicine.)

Side Effects and Contraindications

💣 Opioid administration may be contraindicated in patients with suspected intracranial hypertension unless respiratory monitoring and support is available.

✓ Opioid agonists typically increase vagal tone resulting in a reduced heart rate and in cats may increase body temperature transiently.

✓ Some opioids may cause vomiting and may be contraindicated if an increase in intra-ocular, intra-cranial, intra-abdominal, or esophageal pressure will be detrimental.

✓ Some animals (cats in particular) may become dysphoric following opioid administration. Reduction of dose or co-administration of a tranquilizer will reduce the incidence of dysphoria. Because of interpatient differences in pain tolerance, expect variations in opioid analgesic actions.

Drug Interactions

✓ Opioids have additive or synergistic analgesic effects with alpha$_2$ agonists, NSAIDs, phenothiazines, benzodiazepines, and local anesthetics. Opioids may enhance the respiratory and cardiac depression (e.g., bradycardia) associated with most anesthetic drugs. Cardiopulmonary monitoring should be performed.

Table 2-1 Recommended Opioid Dosages and Indications

Opioid	Dose/Route	Duration (IM)*	Indications	Comments
Morphine	Dog: 0.2 -2.0 mg/kg; IM, SC; 0.05 - 0.4 mg/kg; IV	3 - 5 hr	Moderate to severe pain; CRI at 0.05-0.3 mg/kg/h can be used for long term analgesia	Sedation, respiratory depression, bradycardia, nausea, hypothermia; dysphoria in non-painful cats or with large dosage. To avoid histamine release when given I.V., dilute or administer slowly.
	Cat: 0.05 - 0.2 mg/kg; IM, SC	3 - 4 hr		
Fentanyl	Dog: 0.002 - 0.01 mg/kg; IM, IV, SC	0.5 hr	Moderate to severe pain; CRI at 0.002-0.01 mg/kg/h necessary for long term analgesia	Sedation, respiratory depression, bradycardia, nausea; inadequate duration of analgesia from single IV bolus or IM injection.
	Cat: 0.001 - 0.005 mg/kg; IM, IV, SC	0.5 hr		
Fentanyl Patch	Dog: 0.005 mg/kg/h; Transdermal	3 days	Mild to moderate pain	Onset of effect ranges from 12-24 hours, variability in transdermal absorption may result in inadequate analgesic effects.
	Cat: 0.005 mg/kg/h; Transdermal	3 - 5 days		
Hydromorphone or Oxymorphone	Dog: 0.05 - 0.2 mg/kg; IM, IV, SC	2 - 4 hr	Moderate to severe pain	Similar side effects as those observed with morphine, but less vomiting and no histamine release. Hydromorphone may provide a longer period of analgesia in cats, and has been associated with the occasional observation of hyperthermia in this species.
	Cat: 0.05 - 0.2 mg/kg; IM, IV, SC	2 - 4 hr		
Methadone	Dog: 0.05 - 2.0 mg/kg; PO, IM, SC	4 - 6 hr	Mild to moderate pain	May also have NMDA antagonistic action.
	Cat: 0.05 - 1.0 mg/kg; PO	4 - 6 hr		
Butorphanol	Dog: 0.2 - 2.0 mg/kg; IM IV, SC, PO	1 - 2 hr	Mild to moderate pain	Mild or no sedation, mild ventilatory depression. Butorphanol's analgesic effectiveness in dogs has been debated. Oral bioavailability is uncertain.
	Cat: 0.2 - 1.0 mg/kg; IV, IV, SC, PO	1 - 4 hr		
Buprenorphine	Dog: 0.005 - 0.02 mg/kg; IM, IV, SC	6 - 8 hr	Mild to moderate pain	Onset of analgesic action may require 15-30 min or longer. Prolonged sleep times may occur.
	Cat: 0.005-0.02 mg/kg IM, IV, SC, or transmucosal	6 - 8 hr		Administered orally for absorption through buccal mucosa in cats. May be more difficult to antagonize than other opioid agonists.
		6 - 8 hr		

* Duration varies with dosage and route of administration. Intravenous administration generally results in a more rapid onset and shorter duration, while SC and PO administration usually results in a slower onset and longer duration than listed above for IM administration. Use lower end of dose range for initial IV administration.

Local Anesthetics

Mechanisms of Action

✓ Local anesthetics prevent conduction of nerve impulses by inhibiting passage of sodium ions through ion-selective channels in nerve membranes. Decreased permeability to sodium slows the rate of depolarization so that threshold potential is not achieved and therefore an action potential is not propagated. Stabilization of sodium channels likely occurs in the inactivated-closed state preventing changes in sodium permeability. Sensations disappear in the order of pain, cold, warmth, touch, deep pressure and return in the opposite order. Sensory blockade will usually persist longer than motor blockade (differential block) (See Table 2-2 for dosages and indications of commonly used local anesthetics in veterinary medicine.)

Side Effects and Contraindications

✓ Excessive doses or accidental intravascular injection of local anesthetics may lead to toxic symptoms. Lidocaine may be safely administered intravenously but, at high doses, can cause central nervous system and cardiovascular toxicity. Central nervous system toxic effects include sedation, nausea, ataxia, nystagmus, and tremors. Cardiovascular effects typically follow nervous system toxicity.

✓ Toxic doses of local anesthetics will vary depending on route of administration, coadministered drugs such as epinephrine, site of injection, and species. A general guideline for toxic doses for lidocaine are 10 mg/kg in the dog and 6 mg/kg in the cat. Toxic doses of bupivicaine are lower and are approximately 3.0 mg/kg in the dog and 2.0 mg/kg in the cat.

💣 Bupivacaine can cause cardiovascular toxicity following intravenous administration so this route is contraindicated.

✓ Local anesthetics may cause complete loss of sensation to the body region being treated. A small number of animals may experience anxiety following regional anesthesia (especially epidural). Tranquilization may help in these animals.

✓ When blocking large nerves containing mantle and core bundles, structures innervated by mantel bundles will desensitize first (proximal regions) and structures innervated by core bundles will have delayed blockade of sensation (distal regions).

♥ Dental blocks may cause loss of sensation to the tongue or lips which may result in self-mutilation in some animals.

Table 2-2
Recommended Local Anesthetic Dosages and Indications

LOCAL ANESTHETIC	DOSE/ROUTE	DURATION	INDICATIONS	COMMENTS
Lidocaine (1% to 2% with or without epinephrine)	Dog: up to 6.0 mg/kg; perineural Cat: up to 3.0 mg/kg; perineural	1-2 hr 1-2 hr	All levels of pain	Markedly reduces anesthetic and postoperative analgesic requirements
Lidocaine (constant rate infusion)	Dog: 0.02-0.05 mg/kg/min; IV Cat: 0.01-0.04 mg/kg/min; IV	— —	Mild to moderate chronic pain	Reduces anesthetic and postoperative analgesic requirements; May help to maintain normal GI motility following surgery
Bupivacaine (0.25% to 0.5% with or without epinephrine)	Dog: up to 2.0 mg/kg; perineural Cat: up to 1.0 mg/kg; perineural	2-6 hr 2-6 hr	All levels of pain	Markedly reduces anesthetic and postoperative analgesic requirements
Mepivacaine (1% to 2%)	Dog: up to 6.0 mg/kg; perineural Cat: up to 3.0 mg/kg; perineural	2-2.5 hr 2-2.5 hr	All levels of pain	Markedly reduces anesthetic and postoperative analgesic requirements

The doses given are approximate doses used for a variety of local analgesic/anesthetic techniques. See specific recommended doses under individual techniques in section 3.

Drug Interactions

✓ Local anesthetics can markedly reduce requirements for general anesthetics. Combinations of local anesthetics with opioids have been used for epidural and intra-articular anesthesia, resulting in an enhanced and prolonged duration of hypoalgesia (reduced pain).

✓ Addition of epinephrine (1:200,000) delays absorption and prolongs local anesthetic action.

✓ The addition of 1mEq (1 mL of 8.4% solution) of sodium bicarbonate for every 10 mL of lidocaine will reduce both the discomfort of lidocaine injection and the latency of onset (faster block).

✓ Sodium bicarbonate (1mEq/ml) can cause precipitation if more than 0.5 mL is added to 10 mL of 0.5% bupivicaine.

Alpha$_2$ Adrenergic Agonists

Mechanisms of Action

✓ Alpha$_2$ and opioid receptors are found in similar regions of the brain and even on the same neurons. Both receptor types activate the same signal transduction system mediated by membrane-associated G proteins. Activation of these proteins opens potassium channels, which in turn causes the cell to lose potassium and hyperpolarize. The hyperpolarized cell becomes unresponsive to excitatory input and results in an analgesic or sedative action, depending upon receptor location within the central nervous system. (See Table 2-3 for dosages and indications of commonly used alpha$_2$ agonists in small animal veterinary medicine.)

Side Effects and Contraindications

💣 Use of alpha$_2$ adrenergic agonists may be contraindicated in animals which will be adversely affected by an increase in cardiac afterload or a decrease in cardiac output.

✓ Alpha$_2$ adrenergic agonists increase vagal tone and may cause severe bradycardia.

✔ Duration of analgesic, sedative, and cardiovascular effects are reduced with lower doses of alpha$_2$ agonists.

✔ Vomiting may occur following administration (especially in cats), therefore their use may be contraindicated if an increase in intraocular, intracranial, intra-abdominal, or esophageal pressure will be detrimental.

♥ Alpha$_2$ adrenergic agonists can lead to a transient hypertension and their administration to animals with an increased potential of arterial hemorrhage (e.g., laceration of artery) may be contraindicated.

Table 2-3
Recommended Alpha$_2$ Agonist Dosages and Indications

ALPHA2-AGONIST	DOSE/ROUTE	DURATION (IM)*	INDICATIONS	COMMENTS
Xylazine	Dog: 0.1-0.5 mg/kg; IM, IV	0.5-1.0 hr	Mild pain and/or sedation	Sedation, bradycardia, minimal ventilatory depression, vomiting
	Cat: 0.1-0.5 mg/kg; IM, IV	0.5-1.0 hr		
Medetomidine	Dog: 2-15 µg/kg; IM, IV	0.5-1.5 hr	Mild pain and/or sedation	Coadministration with opioids recommended to enhance analgesic actions. Sedation, bradycardia, minimal ventilatory depression, occasional vomiting
	Cat: 5-20 µg/kg; IM, IV	0.5-1.5 hr		

*Duration varies with dosage and route of administration. IV administration generally results in a more rapid onset and shorter duration than listed above for IM administration. Use low end of dose range for initial IV administration.

Drug Interactions

✔ Alpha$_2$ adrenergic agonists have additive or synergistic effects with opioid analgesic drugs prolonging duration and increasing intensity of effect. Additive and synergistic interactions have also been shown with most anesthetic agents including the inhalants, ketamine, barbiturates, and propofol. Reduced doses of anesthetic are necessary when co-administered with alpha$_2$ adrenergic agonists.

Nonsteroidal Anti-inflammatory Drugs

Mechanisms of Action

✓ Nonsteroidal anti-inflammatory drugs block the first step of prostaglandin synthesis by inhibiting cyclooxygenase enzymes. This inhibition reduces the production of inflammatory mediators known to sensitize peripheral nociceptors. Some newer NSAIDs target the cyclooxygenase enzyme (COX-2) which is presumably responsible for the formation of inducible prostaglandins known to mediate inflammation. They achieve this with minimal effect on the cyclooxygenase enzyme (COX-1) mediating the formation of constitutive prostaglandins important for maintenance of home-ostasis (e.g., normal gastrointestinal, renal, and platelet functions). It is now known that several organ systems rely on COX-2 enzyme activity for mainitance of important functions. Inhibition of the 5-lipoxygenase enzyme has also been targeted as an alternative strategy for managing pain. NSAIDs appear to have a central mechanism of action, although it is poorly understood.

✓ Because pain intensity may wax and wane in an individual patient, NSAID therapy should be customized to reflect chang-ing patient analgesic requirements with the goal of using the minimum effective dose. (See Table 2-4 for dosages and indica-tions of NSAIDs commonly used in veterinary medicine.)

Side Effects, Toxicity, and Contraindications

✓ Cats appear more predisposed to the toxic effects of most NSAIDs, especially with prolonged administration.

💣 Judicious use of NSAIDs is necessary in animals with a history of GI bleeding or renal disease, or in animals being treated concurrently with other drugs known to affect GI or renal function.

✓ It may be prudent to collect baseline biochemistry information before initiating chronic therapy with repeated testing approximately one month later. Once or twice yearly follow-up blood work is recom-mended and all NSAIDs should be titrated down to their minimum effective dose.

✓ Some NSAIDs, most notably aspirin, reduce platelet function leading to prolonged clotting times. These drugs may be contraindicated if bleeding disorders are present or surgery is anticipated in the immediate future.

✓ Lipoxin has been identified as one substance responsible for the adaptation of the GI tract to mucosal injury. Following aspirin therapy, upregulation of lipoxin production via acetylated COX-2 enzyme has been identified as an important mechanism of GI mucosal healing and homeostasis. Following aspirin therapy, caution is recommended when switching to another NSAID capable of inhibiting GI COX-2 enzyme.

Drug Interactions

●※ NSAIDs may enhance the GI and renal toxicity of corticosteroids or other classes of drugs.

✓ Many NSAIDs are highly bound to plasma proteins and may compete with other drugs for binding sites, resulting in increased free-drug concentrations.

✓ NSAIDs may have additive or synergistic drug interactions with opioid agonists resulting in a more intense analgesic effect.

✓ The potential for adverse drug interactions among NSAIDs when administered in sequence is unclear. Recommendations for washout periods when switching between NSAIDs and from glucocorticoid therapy have not been established based upon prospective scientific studies.

✓ A number of medications may be given to reduce the potential for GI pathology when NSAID therapy has been initiated. These include the prostaglandin analogue misoprostol, histamine-2 receptor antagonists such as ranitidine, and proton pump inhibitors such as omeprazole.

✓ Nitric oxide has been incorporated into NSAID preparations and is presently under investigation along with zwitterionic NSAID preparations complexed with phospholipids to help protect the gastrointestinal mucosa.

✓ Because of its well known gastrointestinal side-effects, and the newly recognized potential for adverse interactions if the need to switch to a second NSAID arises, aspirin should not be used as the initial NSAID for peri-operative or chronic pain management.

Table 2-4 Recommended NSAID Dosages and Indications†

NSAIDs	Dosage/Route	Duration (PO)*	Indications	Comments
Carprofen (tablet, chewable and injectable formulations)	Dog: maximum dose of 4.4 mg/kg given once daily or divided into 2 equal doses PO or SC. Injectable approved for SC administration. Cat: 1.0-2.0 mg/kg; once only by injectable route	12-24 hr	Mild to moderate pain; For perioperative soft tissue and orthopedic acute pain and chronic osteoarthritic pain and inflammation in dogs.	Proven minimal toxicity in dogs with long term use. For chronic use titrate to minimum effective dose. When using injectable formulation for preemptive pain control, administration 2 hours prior to surgical incision is recommended. GI upset most common side effect.
Aspirin (tablets)	Dog: 10-25 mg/kg; PO Cat: 10-15 mg/kg; PO	8-12 hr 24-72 hr	Mild to moderate pain and inflammation.	GI irritation, ulcers, kidney damage more likely at higher doses. Contraindicates its use for perioperative pain control.
Etodolac (tablets)	Dog: 10-15 mg/kg; PO Cat: Not Used	24 hr	Mild to moderate arthritis pain in dogs.	Hypoproteinemia, vomiting, loose stools.
Meloxicam (oral liquid suspension and injectable formulations)	Dog: 0.2 mg/kg initially; 0.1 mg/kg thereafter; IM, SC, PO Cat: 0.1 mg/kg initially; 0.025 mg/kg thereafter; IM, SC, PO	24 hr 24 hr	Mild to moderate arthritis pain.	GI irritation; can be mixed with food; use in cats restricted to 2-3 days postoperatively. For chronic arthritic pain in cats reduce dose to 25% short term dose.
Ketoprofen (tablets and injectable)	Dog: 2.0 mg/kg SC, IM initially 1.0 mg/kg thereafter; PO, SC Cat: 1.0 mg/kg SC, IM initially, 0.5 mg/kg thereafter; PO, SC	24 hr 24 hr	Mild to moderate pain.	Increase bleeding time, GI irritation, ulcers, kidney damage reported; not recommended for more than 5 days. May increase bleeding times if given preoperatively.
Deracoxib	Dog: 3.0-4.0 mg/kg for seven days postoperatively and 1.0-2.0 mg/kg for chronic osteoarthritic pain. Cat: Not Used	24 hr	Mild to moderate pain. For acute perioperative orthopedic pain and chronic osteoarthritic pain and inflammation in dogs.	Deracoxib is a member of the coxib class of NSAIDs that possess good cycoolxygenase-2 enzyme selectively. Coxibs may also have antineoplastic actions; GI upset most common side effect.

Drug	Dose	Duration	Indications	Comments
Tepoxalin	Dog: 10-20 mg/kg PO initially; 10 mg/kg thereafter, PO only Cat: Not used	24 hr	Mild to moderate pain. For control of pain and inflammation associated with osteoarthritis in dogs. Preoperative administration is not recommended. When switching from another NSAID to tepoxalin a 7-day washout period is suggested.	Tepoxalin is a dual inhibitor of both cyclooxygenase and lipoxygenase enzyme activity. Formulation is designed to rapidly disintegrate in the mouth. GI upset most common side effect.
Tolfenamic acid (tablets and injectables)	Dog: 4.0 mg/kg SC, IM initially, thereafter PO Cat: same as dog	24 hr 24 hr	Mild to moderate pain.	Vomiting and diarrhea reported; recommended for 4 days on and 3 days off in both dogs and cats.
Acetaminophen (tablets and oral liquid suspension)	Dog: 10-15 mg/kg; PO Cat: Contraindicated	8-12 hr	Mild to moderate pain; low anti-inflammatory action.	**Toxic to cats; Often given in combination with codeine in dogs (see oral analgesic preparations)**

†When toxicity or side effects occur a washout period of several days (5-7) should be observed before reinstating NSAID therapy with an alternative agent.

*Duration varies with routes of administration. IV, IM or SC administration generally results in more rapid onset than that listed for PO administration. In general, following soft tissue injury NSAID therapy is recommended for 3-4 days. Following orthopedic injury NSAIDs are recommended for 7-days or longer. For animals in severe pain combination therapy with opioids may be especially effective.

Analgesic Adjuvant Agents

Mechanism of Action

✓ Adjuvant analgesics have primary medical indications other than pain management, but may provide an hypoalgesic action in some patients. Antidepressants, neuroleptics, corticosteroids, anticonvulsants, sympatholytics, systemic local anesthetics, NMDA receptor antagonists, and central muscle relaxants can all be considered adjuvant analgesics. All of these classes of drugs enhance analgesia by interacting with a variety of receptors or altering nerve conduction processes implicated in pain modulating systems and signal generation or transmission. (See Table 2-5 for dosages and indications for analgesic adjuvant drugs.)

Side Effects and Contraindications

✓ The use of any of the classes of drugs in Table 2-5 is contraindicated where a specific pathophysiologic process is present in which administration would adversely effect the animal's condition.

Drug Interactions

💣 The concomitant use of corticosteroids and NSAIDs, or two or more NSAIDs, may result in an increased risk of developing GI ulcers and nephrotoxicity.

✓ Many adjuvant analgesic drugs alter neurotransmission and conduction processes. Their use in chronic pain conditions may predispose the patient to enhanced effects of other classes of CNS depressant drugs (e.g., general anesthetics). This cautions against the cavalier administration of CNS depressants in patients chronically medicated with adjuvant analgesics.

Table 2-5 Recommended Analgesic Adjuvant Dosages and Indications

ADJUVANT DRUG	DOSE/ROUTE	DURATION (PO)*	INDICATIONS	COMMENTS
Ketamine (NMDA antagonist)	Dog: 0.5 mg/kg; IV 0.1-0.5 mg/kg/hr Cat: 0.5 mg/kg; IV 0.1-0.5 mg/kg/hr CRI	– –	Mild to moderate chronic pain or for analgesia during the postoperative period	Low doses potentiate postoperative analgesics
Acepromazine (phenothiazine)	Dog: 0.025-0.05 mg/kg; IM, SC, IV (maximum total dose: 3 mg) Cat: 0.05-0.2 mg/kg IM, SC	8-12 hr 8-12 hr	Mild to moderate chronic pain and to provide postoperative sedation	Used to potentiate or prolong effects achieved with analgesic drugs
Diazepam (benzodiazepine)	Dog: 0.1-0.2 mg/kg; IV 0.25-1.0 mg/kg; PO Cat: 0.1-0.2 mg/kg; IV 0.25-1.0 mg/kg; PO	2-4 hr 12-24 hr 2-4 hr 12-24 hr	Mild to moderate postoperative or chronic pain	Used to potentiate or prolong analgesia; may be useful adjunctive agent for relieving spastic conditions
Prednisolone (glucocorticoid)	Dog: 0.25-0.5 mg/kg; PO Cat: 0.25-0.5 mg/kg; PO	24-48 hr 24-48 hr	Mild to moderate chronic pain	Use when animals are unresponsive to other analgesic drugs or rapid reduction in inflammation may be life sparing
Amitriptyline (tricyclic antidepressant)	Dog: 1.0 mg/kg; PO Cat: 0.5-1.0 mg/kg; PO	12-24 hr 12-24 hr	Mild to moderate chronic pain	Used to potentiate or prolong analgesia
Tramadol (Opioid agonist)	Dog: 2-10 mg/kg; PO Cat: unknown	12-24 hr –	Moderate to severe chronic pain	Non scheduled oral pain medication; side effects similar to opioids.
Mexilitine (antiarrhythmic)	Dog: 5-10 mg/kg; PO	8-12 hr	Mild to moderate postoperative or chronic pain	Used to potentiate or prolong analgesia
Gabapentin (anticonvulsant)	Dog: 5-10 mg/kg; PO Cat: 5-10 mg/kg; PO	12-24 hr 12-24 hr	Mild to moderate postoperative or chronic pain	Used to potentiate analgesia in patients with neuropathic pain; taper dose when withdrawing drug
Amantidine (NMDA antagonist)	Dog: 3-5 mg/kg; PO Cat: 3-5 mg/kg; PO	24 hr 24 hr	Mild to moderate chronic pain	Neuropathic pain

* Duration varies with dosage and route of administration. IV, IM, and SC administration generally result in a more rapid onset and shorter duration than the duration listed above for PO administration. To select and administer an adjuvant analgesic properly, you should be aware of the drugs clinical pharmacology. The following information about the drug is necessary: 1) approved indication; 2) unapproved indication (e.g., as an analgesic) in veterinary medical practice; 3) common side effects and potentially serious adverse effects; 4) pharmacokinetic features; and 5) specific dosing guidelines for pain.

Preemptive Analgesic Drug Combinations

Several preemptive analgesic drug combinations that are commonly used as preanesthetics in dogs and cats with normal cardiopulmonary function are listed in Figure 2-1. For many short surgical procedures, NSAIDs (e.g., carprofen or deracoxib) may be incorporated with the preanesthetic protocols listed below when contraindications to their use are not present (i.e., preexisting gastrointestinal, renal, or bleeding disorders). For longer surgical procedures, or when compromised tissue perfusion is of concern, NSAID therapy should be delayed until recovery from anesthesia is underway and adequacy of tissue perfusion is assured.

Figure 2-1

MILD PAIN

DOG Midazolam (0.1-0.2 mg/kg) + Butorphanol (0.2-0.4 mg/kg)
ROUTE IM or SC; mixed in same syringe; inject 15-20 minutes before induction of anesthesia

CAT Midazolam (0.05-0.1 mg/kg) + Butorphanol (0.2-0.4 mg/kg)
ROUTE IM or SC; mixed in same syringe; inject 15-20 minutes before induction of anesthesia

DOG Acepromazine (0.025-0.1 mg/kg) + Butorphanol (0.2-0.4 mg/kg)
ROUTE IM or SC; mixed in same syringe; inject 15-20 minutes before induction of anesthesia

CAT Acepromazine (0.025-0.1 mg/kg) + Butorphanol (0.2-0.4 mg/kg)
ROUTE IM or SC; mixed in same syringe; inject 15-20 minutes before induction of anesthesia

DOG Medetomidine (10 micrograms/kg) + Butorphanol (0.2-0.4 mg/kg) + Atropine (0.04 mg/kg)
ROUTE IM or SC; mixed in same syringe; inject 15-20 minutes before induction of anesthesia

CAT Medetomidine (15 micrograms/kg) + Butorphanol (0.2-0.4 mg/kg) + Atropine (0.04 mg/kg)
ROUTE IM or SC; mixed in same syringe; inject 15-20 minutes before induction of anesthesia

DOG Midazolam (0.1-0.2 mg/kg) + Hydromorphone (0.1-0.2 mg/kg)
ROUTE IM or SC; mixed in same syringe; inject 15-20 minutes before induction of anesthesia

CAT Midazolam (0.05-0.1 mg/kg) + Hydromorphone (0.05-0.2 mg/kg)
ROUTE IM or SC; mixed in same syringe; inject 15-20 minutes before induction of anesthesia

DOG Acepromazine (0.05 mg/kg) + Hydromorphone (0.2 mg/kg)
ROUTE IM or SC; mixed in same syringe; inject 15-20 minutes before induction of anesthesia

CAT Acepromazine (0.05 mg/kg) + Hydromorphone (0.05-0.2 mg/kg)
ROUTE IM or SC; mixed in same syringe; inject 15-20 minutes before induction of anesthesia

DOG Acepromazine (0.05 mg/kg) + Morphine (0.5-1.0 mg/kg)
ROUTE IM or SC; mixed in same syringe; inject 15-20 minutes before induction of anesthesia

CAT Acepromazine (0.05 mg/kg) + Morphine (0.1 mg/kg)
ROUTE IM or SC; mixed in same syringe; inject 15-20 minutes before induction of anesthesia

DOG Medetomidine (10 micrograms/kg) + Hydromorphone (0.05-0.2 mg/kg) + Atropine (0.04 mg/kg)
ROUTE IM or SC; mixed in same syringe; inject 15-20 minutes before induction of anesthesia

CAT Medetomidine (15 micrograms/kg) + Hydromorphone (0.05 - 0.2 mg/kg) + Atropine (0.04 mg/kg)
ROUTE IM or SC; mixed in same syringe; inject 15-20 minutes before induction of anesthesia

DOG Medetomidine (10 micrograms/kg) + Morphine (0.5 mg/kg) + Atropine (0.04 mg/kg)
ROUTE IM or SC; mixed in same syringe; inject 15-20 minutes before induction of anesthesia

CAT Medetomidine (15 micrograms/kg) + Morphine (0.1 mg/kg) + Atropine (0.04 mg/kg)
ROUTE IM or SC; mixed in same syringe; inject 15-20 minutes before induction of anesthesia

Note: If heart rates decrease by 30% from awake values, anticholinergic administration is recommended (Atropine 0.02-0.04 mg/kg or Glycopyrrolate 0.005-0.01 mg/kg.)

Transdermal Analgesic Preparations

Fentanyl Patch

✓ Transdermal patches are firmly placed on a clipped region. Patches should be covered with a bandage and applied 12-24 hours before surgery. (See Table 2-6 for recommended patch size for weight of animal.)

✓ Parenteral opioid administration is required immediately following patch application until effective plasma concentrations of fentanyl are established.

Table 2-6
Recommended Fentanyl Patch Sizes

PATIENT	PATCH SIZE
Dog (5 - 10 kg)	25 microgram/hour patch
Dog (10 - 20 kg)	50 microgram/hour patch
Dog (20 - 30 kg)	75 microgram/hour patch
Dog (>30 kg)	100 microgram/hour patch
Cat (2 - 10 kg)	25 microgram/hour patch*

*If cat is small, half of the patch's surface may be covered to reduce dosage of drug.

♥ Analgesic efficacy should be periodically assessed and additional rescue opioids or other analgesics may be required. Variation in absorption, distribution, metabolism, and elimination of fentanyl may vary among patients and even within the same patient following placement of a new patch.

Buprenorphine Patch

✓ Buprenorphine is available in a transdermal matrix patch system which differs slightly from the fentanyl patch system.

✓ Little or no information is available at this time concerning patch characteristics and clinical utility when used in dogs and cats.

✓ Patch sizes include 35, 52.5, and 70 micrograms/h. They are designed to release buprenorphine for up to 72 hours in people.

Information on the duration of drug release and attainment of effective plasma concentrations in dogs and cats is unknown at this time.

Lidocaine Patch

✓ Lidocaine is available for transdermal use in humans to treat peripheral neuropathies such as post-herpetic neuralgia. The use of lidocaine patches is being evaluated in veterinary patients. Anecdotal reports of the use of lidocaine patches for treating chronic neuropathic, post-thoracotomy or ear canal ablation, and mastectomy pain in dogs are encouraging.

✓ In humans, patches are applied for 12 h, then removed for 12 h to minimize the potential for toxicity.

✓ Skin irritation is a reported adverse effect.

✓ Standard Lidoderm patches are 10x14 cm and contain 700 mg of lidocaine in a 5% concentration.

Pluronic Gel Medications

✓ Pluronic gels are compounded formulations containing pluronic copolymer surfactant, active drug, and absorption altering substances such as methylcellulose and soy lecithin. The gels are applied topically under an occlusive bandage to provide a sustained-release topical delivery of analgesic agents such as ketamine, tricyclic antidepressants, and NSAIDs.

✓ Safety and efficacy of these preparations have not been critically assessed but anecdotal evidence suggests they may be beneficial in certain chronic and neuropathic pain syndromes such as facial neuralgia.

✓ Various pluronic gel analgesic preparations are available on request from compounding pharmacies. The efficacy of compounded preparations in transdermal gels is just beginning to be clinically evaluated in dogs and cats.

💣 With few exceptions, the safety and efficacy of compounded analgesic products has not been established. Veterinarians who choose to use pluronic gel preparations should help clients choose a reputable pharmacy and remember that responsibility for safe and effective use of compounded medications delivered via pluronic gels is the veterinarians. Pharmacists have no liability in the event of toxicity or failure of efficacy.

Topical Local Anesthetic Preparations

EMLA Cream

✓ EMLA cream is an eutectic mixture of lidocaine and prilocaine in a ratio of 1:1 by weight. The melting point is below room temperature so both exist as a liquid oil rather than as crystals. It is packaged in 5 gram and 30 gram tubes as well as an anesthetic disc (a single-dose unit of EMLA). The disc contains 1 gram of EMLA emulsion, the active contact surface being approximately 10 cm^2. Each gram of EMLA cream contains lidocaine 25 mg, prilocaine 25 mg, poly-oxyethylene fatty acid esters (as emulsifiers), carboxypolymethylene (as a thickening agent), sodium hydroxide to adjust to a pH of 9, and purified water to a weight of 1 gram.

✓ EMLA cream is used as an analgesic before percutaneous catheterization and superficial minor surgical procedures. The cream should be applied 1 to 2 hours before the anticipated procedure and analgesia will usually last 1 to 2 hours following removal.

✓ EMLA cream may not provide adequate analgesia for procedures involving the deeper subcutaneous structures. Subcutaneous infiltration with a local anesthetic may be necessary.

✓ Application of EMLA cream to broken or inflamed skin may result in increased systemic absorption and toxicity. Application to the middle ear and ocular structures may result in tissue damage. In human infants, EMLA can cause methemoglobinemia. Precautions should be taken to prevent licking or oral ingestion of the cream as passage of the cream through mucous membranes may be greater than through dermal surfaces.

ELA-Max Cream

✓ ELA-Max cream consists of liposomal encapsulated 4% lidocaine preparation. The liposomal preparation allows lidocaine to persist in the epidermis.

✓ This product has been evaluated in cats at a dose of 15 mg/kg applied to clipped skin with no apparent adverse effects. Analgesic effectiveness has not been assessed.

✓ This preparation may be an attractive alternative to EMLA in cats because it does not contain prilocaine which has been associated with methemoglobinemia.

✓ Other local anesthetic preparations effective in producing cutaneous topical analgesia in human patients include tetracaine gel and amethocaine gel formulations that can be applied 45 minutes prior to the initiation of painful procedures.

Dispensable Oral Medications

Some of the oral analgesic preparations that are available for use as dispensable medications for dogs and cats are presented in Tables 2-7, 2-8, and 2-9.

Table 2-7
NSAID Preparations

NSAID	DOG	CAT
Aspirin tablets: 65, 325 mg	10-25 mg/kg PO q 12 hr	10-20 mg/kg PO q 48-72 hr
Carprofen (Rimadyl® tablets: 25, 75, 100 mg or chewables: 25, 75, 100 mg)	2.0 mg/kg PO q 12 hr or 4.4 mg/kg PO q 24 hr	1.0 - 2.0 mg/kg PO q 24 hr (1-2 doses only)
Ketoprofen (Orudis® caplets: 25, 50, 75 mg. In Canada, Anafen® tablets: 5, 20 mg)	2.0 mg/kg PO loading dose, then 1.0 mg/kg q 24 hr (5 days max)	1.0 mg/kg PO loading dose, then 0.05 mg/kg q 24 hr (3 to 5 days max)
Etodolac (Etogesic® tablets: 150, 300 mg)	10-15 mg/kg PO q 24 hr	—
Meloxicam (Metacam® oral suspension: 1.5 mg/ml)	0.2 mg/kg PO loading dose, then 0.1 mg/kg PO q 24 hr	0.1 mg/kg loading dose, then 0.025 mg/kg PO q 24hr (2-3 days)
Acetaminophen tablets: 325, 500 mg, or elixer: 160 mg / 5 ml	15 mg/kg q 8 hr	**Toxic to cats**

Table 2-8
Opioid Preparations

OPIOID	DOG	CAT
Butorphanol (Torbutrol® tablets: 1, 5, 10 mg)	0.2-1.0 mg/kg PO q 1-4 hr	0.2-1.0 mg/kg PO q 4 hr
Codeine tablets: 30, 60 mg	1.0-2.0 mg/kg PO q 6-8 hr	0.1-1.0 mg/kg PO q 4-8 hr
Morphine tablets: 10, 15, 30 mg	0.3-1.0 mg/kg PO q 4-8 hr	—
Morphine (MS Contin® sustained release tablets: 15, 30, 60, 100 mg)	1.5-3.0 mg/kg PO q every 12 hr; Adjust dose as needed	—
Tramadol tablets: 50mg	2-10 mg/kg PO q 12-24; Adjust dose as needed.	—

Table 2-9
Opioid/Acetaminophen Preparations (dog only)

PREPARATIONS	DOG
Codeine 60 mg + Acetaminophen 300 mg (Tylenol® with Codeine #4 tablet)	Dose based on Codeine at 1.0-2.0 mg/kg PO q 6-8 hr
Codeine 2.4 mg/ml + Acetaminophen 24 mg/ml (Tylenol® with Codeine elixir)	Dose based on Codeine at 1.0-2.0 mg/kg PO q 6-8 hr
Oxycodone 5 mg + Acetaminophen 325 mg (Percocet® tablet)	Dose based on Acetaminophen at 10-15 mg/kg PO q 8-12 hr

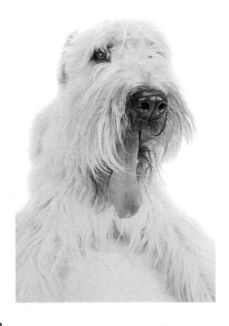

Section 3

Analgesic Techniques

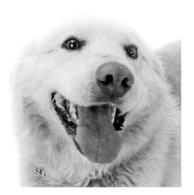

Epidural Analgesia/Anesthesia

Technique

Patients are typically sedated or anesthetized and placed in sternal or lateral recumbency. Sternal recumbency facilitates the hanging drop technique whereas lateral recumbency facilitates positioning of animals with fractures. Next, the cranial edge of the wings of the ilia are palpated. A line connecting these two points typically overlies the vertebral body of L7. Just caudal to this line, an indentation can be felt which corresponds to the lumbosacral junction. Location can be verified by palpating the dorsal spinous process of the seventh lumbar vertebra rostral to this indentation. Once located, a 10 cm by 10 cm area of hair directly over the lumbosacral junction is clipped and the skin is surgically prepared. Needle insertion is made directly over the depression formed by the lumbosacral junction with the needle initially positioned perpendicular to the skin. It is important the stylet is correctly positioned within the needle to prevent transplantation of skin into the epidural space.

When using the hanging drop technique, the stylet is removed after penetrating the skin and placed on a sterile area (typically the paper glove liner). Then a few drops of solution are placed in the hub of the needle until a meniscus is formed. The needle is slowly advanced until it encounters bone or punctures the ligamentum flavum. If bone is struck the needle is withdrawn to the subcutaneous tissue and redirected. If the ligamentum flavum is punctured and the needle tip enters the epidural space, fluid will typically flow from the hub of the needle into the space (Figure 3-1).

If the epidural is being performed while the animal is in lateral recumbency, the stylet is left in the needle until a characteristic pop is felt as the ligamentum flavum is punctured.

With both techniques, following insertion and removal of the stylet, the needle is observed for flow of cerebral spinal fluid or blood.

Once the tip of the needle is confirmed to be in the epidural space, the syringe is attached to the hub of the epidural needle and a slow injection of the analgesic agent is begun. Observation of the lack of compression of a small (1 ml) air bubble in the syringe helps to ensure that there is no resistance to injection.

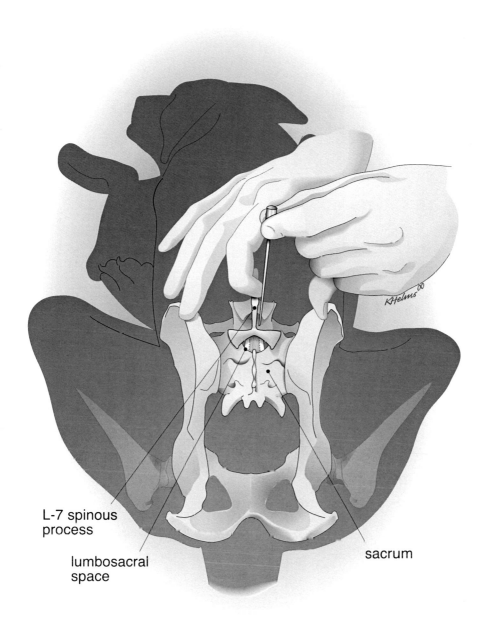

L-7 spinous
process

lumbosacral
space

sacrum

Figure 3-1
Anatomic landmarks for epidural technique

Following injection the needle is withdrawn and the surgical site is placed ventrally in order to facilitate the movement of analgesic drug to the correct side of the spinal cord. Other signs indicating correct needle placement may include twitching of the tail muscles and a change of respiratory pattern during injection. If blood flows out of the needle, it can be withdrawn and flushed, then reinserted (with the stylet in place). If cerebrospinal fluid flows out of the needle and the decision is made to inject analgesic into the subarachnoid space, the dose volume should be reduced by at least 50%.

Materials Needed

Spinal needle - Quincke or Huber point 22-18 gauge
1.5 to 2.5 inch sterile syringe
Sterile gloves

Drugs and Dosages

Lidocaine (2%) or bupivacaine (0.25%-0.5%) with or without epinephrine. Dose is 1 ml / 4.5 kg for caudal procedures or 1 ml / 3.5 kg for abdominal procedures. Duration is prolonged 1.0 to 1.5 hours when combined with epinephrine. When diluting drugs with saline or local anesthetic, keep the total epidural injection volume below 0.25 ml/kg. Lidocaine provides 1-3 hours, while bupivacaine provides 4-6 hours of analgesia.

Morphine (15 mg/ml); (0.1 mg/kg combined with 1.0 ml of saline or local anesthetic / 4.5 kg body weight).

Preservative-free morphine (1.0 mg/ml); (0.1-0.3 mg/kg); a 0.2 mg/kg dose is equal to a volume of about 1.0 ml / 4.5 kg body weight undiluted. Morphine may result in 6-12 h of analgesia when given alone and much longer when coadministered with a local anesthetic.

Preservative-free fentanyl (50 micrograms/ml); 5-10 micrograms/kg, in the dog.

Preservative-free buprenorphine (300 micrograms/ml); 5-20 micrograms/kg, in the dog, 5-10 micrograms/kg, in the cat.

Local anesthetics and morphine are commonly combined at the above dosages to enhance epidural analgesia.

Complications and Contraindications

♥ Sterile technique is mandatory.

♠※ Inflammation, coagulopathy, or other pathology in the area of the lumbosacral junction may be a contraindication to epidural drug placement.

♠※ Local anesthetic solutions should not be administered epidurally or spinally to patients at risk for hypotension because inhibition of sympathetic efferent activity may cause vasodilation.

✓ Urinary retention may occur following epidural injection of local anesthetics and opioids. Patients should be periodically assessed for bladder distention.

Technical Skill

✓ This procedure requires moderate skill. Difficulty varies with body condition and size of animal.

⊙ See CD for demonstration of Epidural Analgesia/Anesthesia technique (Video 3-1).

Epidural Catheter Placement

Technique

If radiographic verification of the placement of the catheter is desired, the patient should be sedated or anesthetized and the procedure performed on the table top of an X-ray machine. A mask, hair covering, and two pairs of sterile gloves should be worn. Location of landmarks and preparation of the area are similar to that described for the epidural technique, although a wider surgical clip and prep to facilitate sterile introduction of the catheter is advocated. Following preparation, the animal is draped so only a small area of skin is exposed over the lumbosacral space. A Touhy needle is introduced through the skin and directed toward the lumbosacral junction. The needle should be directed cranioventrally rather than perpendicularly to facilitate passage of the catheter. (See Figure 3-2.)

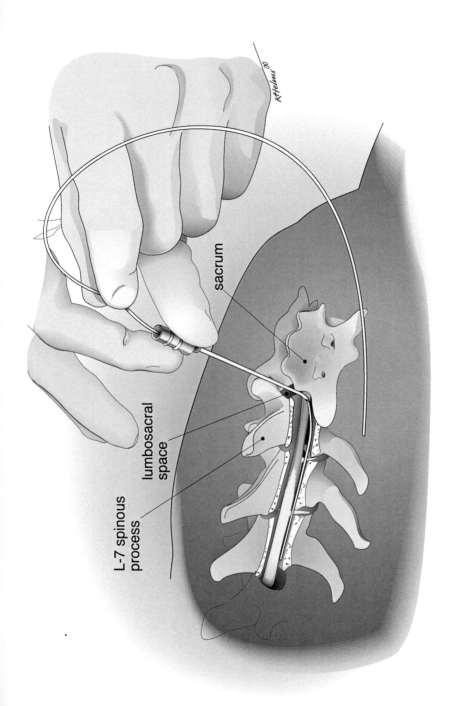

sacrum

lumbosacral space

L-7 spinous process

Figure 3-2

Anatomic landmarks for epidural catheter placement

Once the needle is in the lumbosacral epidural space, the stylet is removed and a small test injection of sterile saline can be made to confirm positioning. Next, the outer pair of gloves are removed and discarded before the catheter is handled. The length of catheter needed is estimated by measuring the distance from the lumbosacral space rostrally to the desired site of action on the spinal cord and nerves, allowing for the distance from skin to spinal canal, and some extra length for later positioning. The catheter is then gently placed through the needle into the epidural space. Some slight resistance may be felt. The catheter should not be forced. NEVER withdraw the catheter back through the needle; this may shear off the catheter in the epidural space.

When the desired positioning is achieved, a radiograph may be taken to confirm placement. If the catheter does not have a wire stylet, a small injection of radiographic contrast media may facilitate visualization of the catheter. Once proper positioning is achieved, the wire stylet is removed and the Touhy needle is withdrawn. Next, the adapter is positioned on the proximal end of the catheter. Gentle aspiration at this point may identify inadvertent catheter placement in a venous sinus or the subarachnoid space.

The filter and injection cap are pre-assembled and charged with saline or epidural drug solution to remove air. Then the assembly is attached to the adapter. If the catheter is to be left in place for more than a few days, two filters may be used. The first filter can be changed periodically, but the second can be left undisturbed to keep the interior of the catheter sterile. The whole assembly is then sutured in place. Bandaging may be attempted but it may be difficult to maintain (especially in male dogs). An Elizabethan collar is also recommended if the animal is likely to chew at the catheter. Any future handling of the open catheter or injections into the catheter should be done sterilely. It may be prudent to culture the tip of the catheter when it is removed even if there are no signs of infection.

Materials Needed

Epidural catheter
Touhy needle
Catheter adapter
0.2 micron filters
Injection cap
Sterile syringe with saline, sterile gloves and drape
Towel clamps

Needle holder
Sterile syringe with analgesic drugs
2-0 nylon suture
Bandage materials

Many of these items may be purchased prepackaged in epidural catheter trays, or the catheter, needle, and adapter may be purchased in a more economical epidural kit. Two sizes are generally available; adult size with a 17 gauge x 3 in. needle and 19 gauge catheter and stylet, or a pediatric size with a 20 gauge x 2 in. needle and 24 gauge x 75 cm catheter.

Drugs and Dosages

Use preservative-free morphine (1 mg/ml) 0.1-0.2 mg/kg every 8 hours or 0.3-0.5 mg/kg/day as a CRI. Morphine is less lipophilic and diffuses throughout the epidural space, potentially providing analgesia as far cranial as the cervical spinal cord.

Preservative-free fentanyl (50 micrograms/ml) 1-5 micrograms/kg/h as a CRI in dogs. Fentanyl is more lipophilic than morphine and will remain localized in the region of the catheter tip.

Preservative-free buprenorphine (300 micrograms/ml) 5-20 micrograms/kg every 8 hours or 15-60 micrograms/kg/day as a CRI in dogs or cats. Buprenorphine is similar to fentanyl with regard to its local site of action.

Preservative-free bupivacaine (0.0625%-0.125%); 1 ml/4.5 kg followed by 0.1-0.4 ml/kg/h as a CRI. Reduced concentrations of bupivacaine will lessen motor nerve blockade. Do not exceed 4 mg/kg/day in dogs.

Volume and rate of injection will also influence drug distribution within the epidural space.

Complications and Contraindications

♥ Migration of local anesthetic to the cranial thoracic or cervical spinal cord can cause motor blockade to the respiratory muscles and block sympathetic nerves responsible for regulation of cardiovascular function.

💣 Repeated injection of drugs which contain preservatives may result in damage to the spinal cord and neurological dysfunction.

✔ The same complications and contraindications apply as for epidural drug administration with the addition of possible hind limb weakness and prolonged urinary retention.

✔ It is important to reposition the animals every 2 to 4 hours since normal sensation to a significant part of the body may be reduced or absent. Prolonged pressure on nerves and muscles may result in temporary or permanent dysfunction.

✔ The risk of serious infection will usually increase over time. Therefore the catheter should be removed as soon as it is no longer needed.

● Aseptic technique is essential for placement of the catheter and for handling during subsequent injections.

Technical Skill

✔ This procedure requires a high level of skill.

◉ See CD for demonstration of Epidural Catheter Placement technique (Video 3-2).

Brachial Plexus Block

Technique

Anatomic landmarks are the point of the shoulder, the first rib, and the transverse processes of the cervical vertebrae (Figure 3-3). An area cranial and dorsal to the point of the shoulder is clipped and prepared with surgical scrub. This is often done during the preparation of the leg for surgery. With the neck in a natural position, the cervical transverse processes will form a line which if continued, will usually traverse the proximal brachial plexus. An alternative method is to insert the needle proximal to the point of the shoulder. Using either approach, the needle should be inserted until the tip is just caudal to the first rib. Keep the needle guided beneath the scapula but outside the thorax. Then the syringe is attached and aspiration is attempted to check for accidental puncture of a blood vessel. After confirmation of correct needle placement, 1 or 2 ml of the analgesic solution is injected. Then the needle is withdrawn approximately 1 cm, and the process of aspirating and injecting is repeated until the needle is just ready to exit the skin. It is often difficult to assess the efficacy of the block until after the effects of the general anesthetic have worn off. The block may be repeated before awaking the animal if the surgical procedure was long.

A second technique utilizing an insulated locator needle can be used to help with accurate needle placement and reduce local anesthetic dose requirements. One lead from the nerve stimulator is attached to the skin and the other to the proximal portion of the needle. The needle is passed caudal to the surface of the first rib as described above. As the needle is inserted, the highest current setting is on and as the paw begins to twitch, the needle is positioned to induce the maximal twitch with the least current possible. Local anesthetic is then injected until the twitch stops. Usually a small volume will be effective. This is repeated above and below this site to ensure entire plexus blockade.

Materials Needed

A 22 gauge 2 to 3 inch spinal needle or catheter stylet will work well for the blind technique.
A 22 gauge 3 inch insulated needle for the locater needle technique.
Sterile syringe

Drugs and Dosages

Bupivacaine (0.5%); approximately 1 ml / 4.5 kg. Lidocaine (2%); approximately 1 ml / 4.5 kg.

Do not exceed the toxic dose recommendation of either local anesthetic.

Complications and Contraindications

✓ Brachial plexus blocks are relatively safe and easy to perform. Guard against an accidental insertion of needle tip into the thoracic cavity or a blood vessel.

✓ Contraindications include infection in the nearby tissues or history of sensitivity to the drugs being used.

Technical Skill

✓ This procedure requires minimal skill.

◉ See CD for demonstration of Brachial Plexus Block technique (Video 3-3).

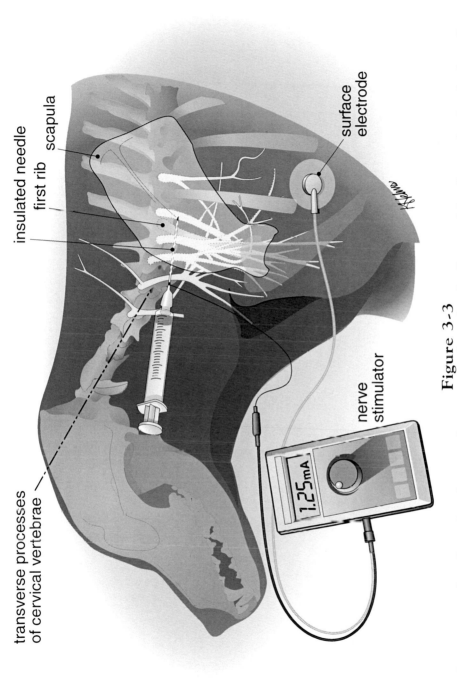

Figure 3-3

Anatomic landmarks for performing a brachial plexus block with the help of a Nerve Locator.

Radial/Ulnar/Median Nerve Block

Proximal Technique

The forelimb is clipped on the medial and lateral aspect from above the elbow to the shoulder. The skin is prepped in the mid diaphyseal region on the medial and lateral aspects. The median and ulnar nerves can be palpated at the point of bifurcation just caudomedial to the mid humerus. Local anesthetic, 0.5 to 1.5 ml, can be deposited around the nerves at this site. Blockade of the median and ulnar nerve should desensitize the medial and caudal/palmar aspect of the antebrachium and paw. The radial nerve can be palpated on the caudo-lateral aspect of the mid humerus opposite the median and ulnar nerves. The nerve can usually be palpated at this level. Local anesthetic, 0.5 to 1.5 ml, can be deposited at this site. Blockade of the radial nerve should desensitize the cranial/dorsal and lateral aspects of the antebrachium and paw.

Distal Technique

The superficial branches of the radial nerve, the median nerve, and the dorsal and palmar branches of the ulnar nerve can be blocked more distally by placing 0.1 to 0.3 ml of local anesthetic at each of three locations. The median nerve and palmar branch of the ulnar nerve can be blocked medial to the accessory carpal pad; the dorsal branch of the ulnar nerve can be blocked lateral and proximal to the accessory carpal pad; finally, the superficial branches of the radial nerve can be blocked at the dorso-medial aspect of the proximal carpus (Figure 3-4).

Materials Needed

20 or 22 gauge hypodermic needle
Sterile syringe

Radial/Ulnar/Median Nerve Block (Distal)

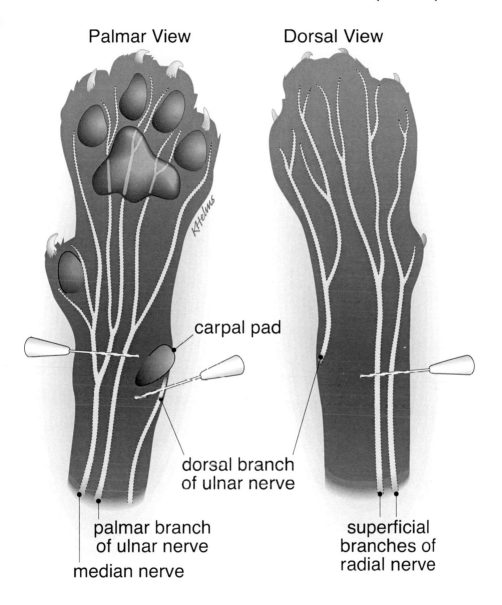

Palmar View

Dorsal View

carpal pad

dorsal branch
of ulnar nerve

palmar branch
of ulnar nerve

median nerve

superficial
branches of
radial nerve

Figure 3-4
Distal radial/ulnar/median nerve blocks

Drugs and Dosages

Proximal Block

Lidocaine (2%) with or without epinephrine; 0.5 to 1.5 ml per injection site not to exceed toxic dose.

Bupivacaine (0.5%) with or without epinephrine; 0.5 to 1.5 ml per injection site not to exceed toxic dose.

Distal Block

Lidocaine (2%); 0.1 to 0.3 ml per injection site

Bupivacaine (0.5%); 0.1 to 0.3 ml per injection site

Complications and Contraindications

✓ Infection at the injection site may be a contraindication for median/ulnar nerve blocks.

💣 Although extremely rare animals should be observed for signs of self-mutilation following recovery.

Technical Skill

✓ This procedure requires minimal skill.

◉ See CD for demonstration of Radial/Ulnar/Median Nerve Block (Video 3-4).

Intra-articular Analgesia

Technique

The procedure is typically performed following exploration of a joint but it can be performed preemptively. The area over the joint to be injected is clipped and surgically prepared (may be done during the surgical preparation). The anatomic landmarks used for locating the joint space will vary depending on the joint being injected. This technique is most commonly employed for stifle arthrotomy. The landmarks for deposition into the stifle are the lateral femoral condyle, the lateral aspect of the tibial tuberosity, patellar ligament, and patella (Figure 3-5). This technique should be performed in a sterile fashion. The needle will penetrate skin, subcutaneous tissue, and joint capsule and should be directed caudo-medially to enter the joint immediately lateral and distal to the distal tip of the patella. If injection is done during surgery, direct visualization of the joint capsule will help with location. The needle is inserted and joint fluid is allowed to flow out of the joint. The analgesic/anesthetic solution is then injected until the desired volume is delivered (usually slight distention of the joint capsule corresponds to correct volume).

Materials Needed

22 gauge sterile hypodermic needle
Sterile syringe

Drugs and Dosages

Lidocaine (2%); a volume up to 1 ml / 4.5 kg (may be better choice over bupivacaine if used preemptively because of faster onset).

Bupivacaine (0.5%); a volume up to 1 ml / 4.5 kg

Morphine (15 mg/ml); 0.1-0.3 mg/kg; opioids appear to be more efficacious in chronically inflamed joints.

Complications and Contraindications

✓ Injections of infected joints may be contraindicated.

💣 If sterile technique is not used or contaminated drug solutions are injected, septic arthritis may develop.

Technical Skill

This procedure requires minimal skill. Intra-articular anesthesia may be a good alternative to epidural anesthesia for procedures of the stifle or other joints.

⦿ See CD for demonstration of Intra-articular Analgesia technique (Video 3-5).

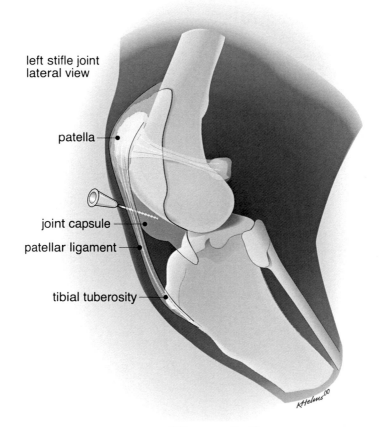

left stifle joint
lateral view

patella

joint capsule

patellar ligament

tibial tuberosity

Figure 3-5
Anatomic landmarks for intra-articular injection

Dental Nerve Blocks

Technique

Dental blocks are typically performed while the animal is anesthetized.

Infraorbital Nerve Block

Several branches of the infraorbital nerve supply sensory innervation to the upper dental arcade (Figure 3-6A). The caudal maxillary alveolar nerve branches off the infraorbital nerve just as it enters the maxillary foramen and supplies the caudal maxillary teeth. Within the infraorbital canal the middle maxillary alveolar nerve branches to supply the middle maxillary teeth. The rostral maxillary alveolar nerve branches off the infraorbital nerve just prior to its exit from the infraorbital canal. This branch supplies innervation to the upper canine teeth and incisors. The infraorbital artery and vein travel with the infraorbital nerve within the canal and should be avoided when injecting analgesic solution.

Blocking the rostral branches of the infraorbital nerve (rostral maxillary nerve): the infraorbital foramen is palpated through the buccal mucosa dorsal to the upper third premolar. Blockade of the nerve at this point will provide anesthesia to the ipsilateral canine teeth and incisors. The needle is inserted to just inside the infraorbital foramen. Aspiration is attempted before injection to ascertain if the needle has inadvertently entered a vessel. Then 0.25-0.5 ml of local anesthetic is injected.

Blocking the caudal and middle branches of the infraorbital nerve (caudal and middle maxillary alveolar nerves): the infraorbital foramen is palpated above the third upper premolar. The length of the infraorbital canal is estimated by palpating the caudal ventral margin of the bony orbit. A 22 or 25 gauge needle is inserted into the infraorbital canal in a caudal-dorsal direction while holding the syringe parallel to the long axis of the jaw. The needle should advance without much resistance to the predetermined depth. After aspiration, 0.25-0.5 ml of local anesthetic is slowly injected.

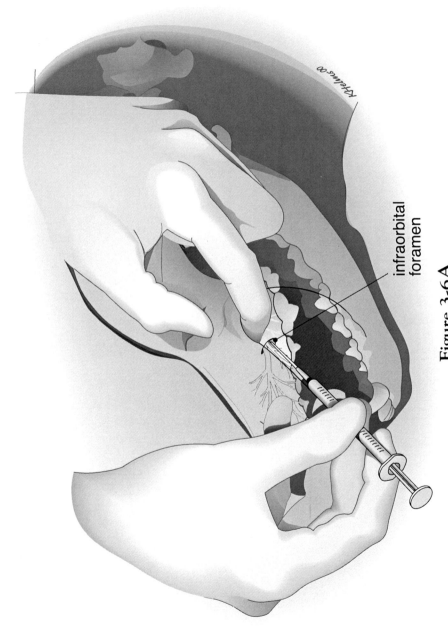

infraorbital
foramen

Figure 3-6A
Anatomic landmarks for performing infraorbital nerve blocks

Mandibular Nerve Block

The mandibular nerve is a branch of the trigeminal nerve and provides sensory innervation to the mandibular teeth (Figure 3-6B). The nerve enters the mandibular foramen on the medial aspect of the mandible just rostral to the angle of the mandible. The foramen is easily palpated from inside the mouth just caudal to the last molar. It is sometimes easier to palpate the nerve under the mucosa and follow it to the mandibular foramen. Blockade at this level provides analgesia to the teeth of the ipsilateral mandible.

Trans-oral approach: use a 25 gauge needle attached to a tuberculin syringe to draw up 0.25-1.0 ml of local anesthetic. Palpate the mandibular foramen with the index finger of one hand and introduce the syringe with the other. Once the tip of the needle is palpated next to the foramen, aspiration is attempted and the anesthetic can be injected.

Transcutaneous approach: a small area of skin ventro-medial to the angle of the mandible is clipped and prepped. A 22 or 25 gauge needle is attached to a tuberculin syringe and 0.25-1.0 ml of local anesthetic is drawn up. The mandibular foramen is transorally palpated with the index finger of one hand while the needle is introduced through the skin with the other. The needle is directed to the mandibular foramen by palpation and when in the proper position, aspiration is attempted and injection of the anesthetic is completed.

Materials Needed

Tuberculin syringe
22 or 25 gauge needle

Drugs and Dosages

Lidocaine (2.0%); 0.25-1.0 ml per site. Dose selection depends on the size of the animal. If multiple sites are to be blocked, keep total dose below the toxic level for that species.

Bupivacaine (0.5%); 0.25-1.0 ml per site. Dose selection depends on the size of the animal. If multiple sites are to be blocked, keep total dose below the toxic level for that species.

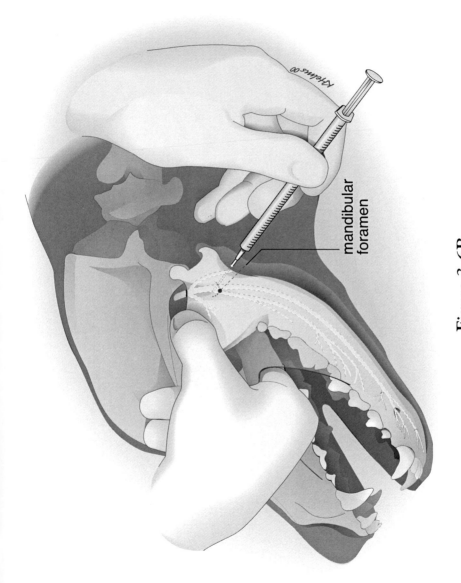

mandibular
foramen

Figure 3-6B
Anatomic landmarks for performing mandibular dental nerve blocks

Complications and Contraindications

✓ Injection into infected tissue is contraindicated.

💣※ Animals may be at risk for self-mutilation following sensory loss to the tongue or lips.

✓ Tranquilization may be required in a small percentage of animals to offset anxiety induced by loss of sensation to the mouth.

Technical Skill

✓ This procedure requires moderate skill.

◉ See CD for demonstration of Dental Nerve Block techniques (Video 3-6).

Infiltrative Blocks

Technique

The hair over the area to be desensitized is clipped and the skin is surgically prepared. The smallest size needle should be used. An inverted pyramid is envisioned beneath the area to be desensitized. This area should be infiltrated to assure blockade of sensory nerve endings around and below the lesion. The needle is introduced in one of the corners of the base of the triangle. Local anesthetic is injected as the needle is directed along one side of the pyramid. The needle is then withdrawn to the subcutaneous tissue and redirected along an adjacent side of the pyramid. Again, anesthetic is injected. Next, the needle is withdrawn and reinserted through an area of desensitized skin from the previous injections. This technique minimizes the number of needle insertions into sensitive skin. This is repeated until all of sides of the pyramid, to its apex, have been infiltrated, creating an area of skin and subcutaneous tissue that is completely desensitized (Figure 3-7). Epinephrine (1:200,000) may be used to reduce systemic absorption of the local anesthetic thus prolonging analgesia. Epinephrine should not be used in tissues sites where intense vasoconstriction of vessels can lead to ischemia.

When long term infiltrative analgesia is desired such as following ear canal ablation, amputation, or thoracotomy, an implantable catheter attached to a disposable elastomeric reservoir (PainBuster Soaker®) may be used. The fenestrated catheter is placed in the surgical site. Following surgery, the reservoir is filled with local anesthetic solution and can be set to deliver a constant rate of 0.5 to 5 mL/h up to 5 days. Preliminary studies in canine patients have shown this device to be effective (See Figure 4-1).

Materials Needed
Sterile hypodermic needle, 22 or 25 gauge
Sterile syringe

Drugs and Dosages
Total dose should be less than toxic dose.

Single injection doses:

Lidocaine (2.0%) with or without epinephrine:
Dogs; < 6.0 mg/kg.
Cats; < 3.0 mg/kg.

Bupivacaine (0.5%) with or without epinephrine:
Dogs; < 2.0 mg/kg.
Cats; < 1.0 mg/kg.

A 1:1 mixture of lidocaine and bupivacaine may be used to achieve a rapid onset and longer duration of blockade.

Total dose when co-administered should not exceed 3.0 mg/kg of lidocaine and 2.0 mg/kg of bupivacaine.

Continuous local infusion with devices like the Pain Buster, allows for variation in the rate of administration. Dilution of the local anesthetic may be required to avoid toxicity.

Figure 3-7
Infiltrative anesthesia/analgesia

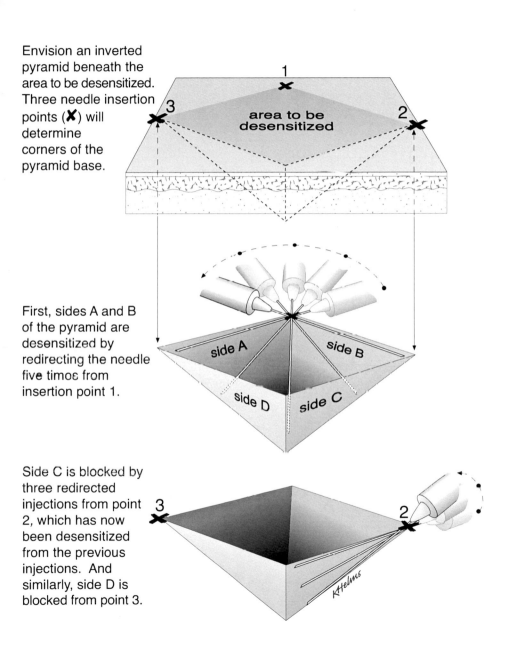

Envision an inverted pyramid beneath the area to be desensitized. Three needle insertion points (✗) will determine corners of the pyramid base.

1

3

area to be desensitized

2

First, sides A and B of the pyramid are desensitized by redirecting the needle five times from insertion point 1.

side A   side B

side D   side C

Side C is blocked by three redirected injections from point 2, which has now been desensitized from the previous injections. And similarly, side D is blocked from point 3.

3

2

KHelms

Complications and Contraindications

✓ Possible complications include inadvertent intravenous or intra-arterial injection, penetration of body cavities or organs, or allergic reactions to the injected drugs (rare).

✓ Infiltrative anesthesia may cause excessive bleeding due to vasodilation caused by sympathetic blockade to the small vessels. This can be reduced by using solutions containing epinephrine.

💣 In smaller patients be sure not to exceed toxic doses.

Technical Skill

✓ This procedure requires minimal skill.

⊙ See CD for demonstration of Infiltrative Block technique (Video 3-7)

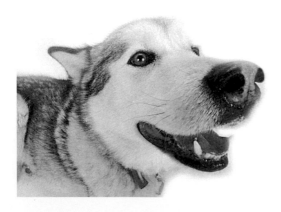

Intravenous Regional Analgesia/Anesthesia

Technique

First an intravenous catheter is placed in an appropriate and accessible vein (usually the cephalic or saphenous vein, or a branch thereof) distal to the proposed tourniquet site. The limb is then desanguinated by wrapping it with an Esmarch bandage; the elastic bandaging material begins at the distal aspect of the limb and is wrapped tightly in a proximal direction. A tourniquet is then placed immediately proximal to the Esmarch bandage. The tourniquet must be tight enough to overcome arterial blood pressure. After securing the tourniquet, the Esmarch bandage is removed and the drug is injected intravenously with light pressure. Maximal anesthesia is achieved in 5 to 10 minutes (Figure 3-8). A second tourniquet can be placed distal to the first tourniquet once blockade has occurred allowing for release of pressure over the original site of tissue compression. Continued occlusion of vessels in an area of the limb that has already been desensitized often reduces the level of tourniquet pain experienced by the patient.

Materials Needed

Bandage material (e.g., Vetrap) for Esmarch bandage
Intravenous catheter
Tourniquet
Sterile syringe
Sterile needle

Drugs and Dosages

Lidocaine (2.0%); 2.5-5.0 mg/kg in the dog.

💣 Do not use bupivacaine for intravenous regional anesthesia because of its potential cardiotoxicity when given by this route.

Total volume injected will depend upon the size of the area that is occluded by the tourniquet.

The tourniquet should be removed slowly to avoid rapid introduction of a large volume of lidocaine into the systemic circulation.

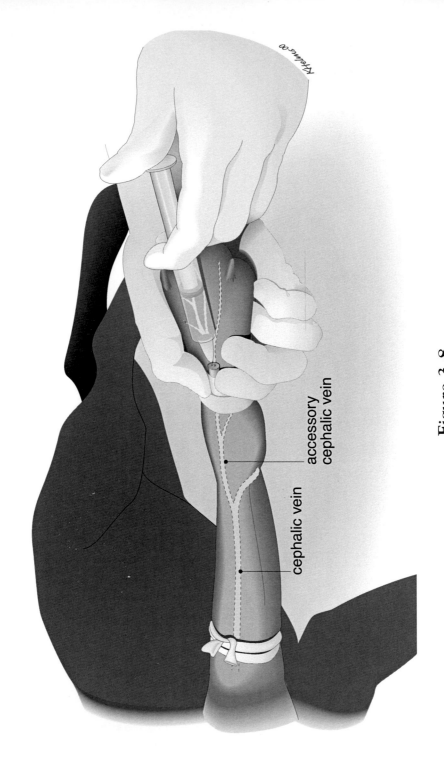

accessory
cephalic vein

cephalic vein

Figure 3-8
Intravenous regional anesthesia/analgesia of the forelimb

Complications and Contraindications

💣※ Ischemic limb damage can occur if tourniquet is in place for more than 90 minutes.

✓ Symptoms of systemic local anesthetic toxicity may occur if tourniquet is not tight enough or released rapidly.

Technical Skill

✓ This procedure requires moderate skill.

⊙ See CD for demonstration of Intravenous Regional Analgesia/Anesthesia technique (Video 3-8).

Intercostal Nerve Block

Technique

Intercostal nerve blocks can be performed prior to surgery or intra-operatively, either during or after thoracotomy. A minimum of 2 adjacent intercostal spaces both cranial and caudal to the incision or injury site must be blocked due to overlapping nerve supply. The needle is introduced percutaneously, using aseptic technique, at the caudal border of the rib near the level of the intervertebral foramen (Figure 3-9). The needle should penetrate skin, subcutaneous tissue, and then intercostal muscles before the appropriate volume of local anesthetic is deposited. Post-thoracotomy pain is generally controlled for 3 to 6 hours following successful block.

Materials Needed

Sterile syringe
Sterile needle

Drugs and Dosages

Lidocaine (2.0%); 0.25-1.0 ml per site. Dose selection depends on the size of the animal. If multiple nerves are to be blocked, keep total dose below the toxic level.

Bupivacaine (0.5%); 0.25-1.0 ml per site. Dose selection depends on the size of the animal. If multiple nerves are to be blocked, keep total dose below the toxic level.

Complications and Contraindications

♥ Intrathoracic injection with the possibility of pneumothorax or pulmonary laceration.

✓ Slight risk of systemic local anesthetic toxicity.

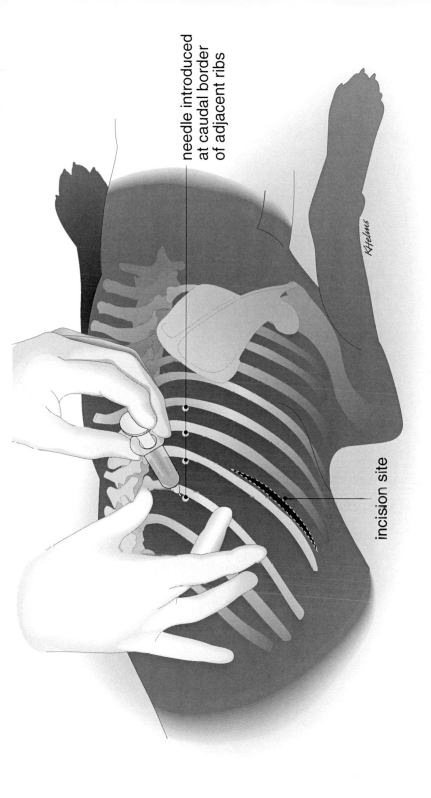

needle introduced
at caudal border
of adjacent ribs

incision site

KHelms

Figure 3-9
Anatomic landmarks for intercostal nerve block

62

Technical Skill

✓ This procedure requires moderate skill.

⊙ See CD for demonstration of Intercostal Nerve Block technique (Video 3-9).

Interpleural Intraperitoneal Intraincisional Analgesia/Anesthesia

Technique

The procedure is done with the animal either heavily sedated or anesthetized at the end of a thoracotomy. Chest tubes are placed in animals that would benefit from interpleural anesthesia following surgery. If a chest tube is not being placed, a commercially available interpleural anesthesia tray may be used. The technique requires desensitization of the skin, subcutaneous tissue, and parietal pleura by infiltration of 2% lidocaine. An intravenous catheter or Touhy needle is then used for interpleural catheter placement. Following skin penetration with the needle, the stylet is removed and the needle filled with sterile saline until a hanging drop is seen on the hub of the needle. The needle is then advanced between the ribs until a clicking sensation is felt as the needle tip penetrates the parietal pleura or until the hanging drop is sucked into the needle by negative pressure generated within the pleural space upon inspiration (Figure 3-10). The catheter is then introduced into the interpleural space through the needle and advanced several centimeters or until resistance is encountered. The needle is removed and the adapter is attached to the end of the catheter. Prior to injection of local anesthetic, the catheter should be aspirated for air or blood. Then the analgesic solution is injected and the catheter cleared with 1.0 to 2.0 ml of air or saline solution, closed to room air, and secured to the thoracic wall. The animal is then positioned to facilitate fluid movement to the area of tissue damage. Take care to prevent inadvertent pneumothorax during

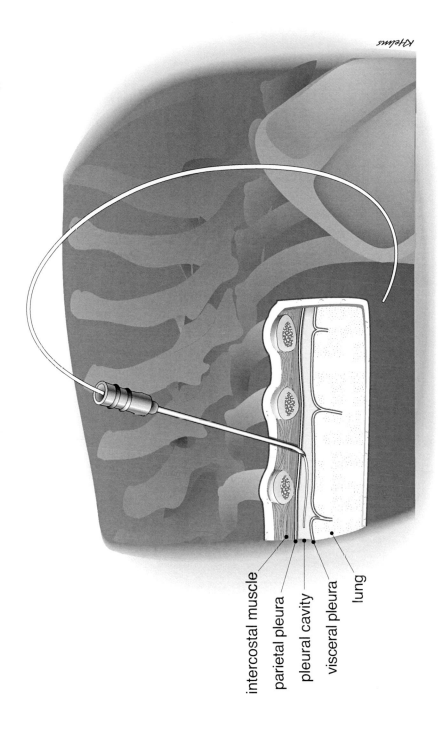

intercostal muscle
parietal pleura
pleural cavity
visceral pleura
lung

Figure 3-10
Anatomic landmarks for interpleural analgesia/anesthesia

64

catheter placement or anesthetic injection. After injection of the local anesthetic the chest tube is not aspirated for 60 minutes unless the animal appears to be experiencing respiratory distress associated with pneumo- or hemothorax.

Intraperitoneal/incisional infusion is commonly performed under anesthesia at the end of an abdominal surgery (OHE, exploratory laparotomy). Before skin closure the solution of local anesthetic is infused through the cranial portion of the incision into the abdominal cavity. After the linea alba is sutured, an additional 2 ml of undiluted solution can be dripped onto the subcutaneous tissues prior to skin closure. During recovery, the animal can be placed in sternal recumbency for approximately 10 minutes to allow the local anesthetic to make contact with the incision site.

Materials Needed

Chest tube or interpleural catheter tray
Sterile gloves
Sterile needle
Sterile syringe

Drugs and Dosages

Interpleural Block

Lidocaine (2.0% without epinephrine):
Dogs; < 6.0 mg/kg every 2 to 4 hrs.
Cats; < 3.0 mg/kg every 4 hrs.

Bupivacaine (0.25% without epinephrine):
Dogs; < 2.0 mg/kg initial dose, then 1.0 mg/kg every 6 hrs.
Cats; < 1.0 mg/kg initial dose, then 0.5 mg/kg every 6 hrs.

Saline solution (5 - 20 ml) may be used to increase injection volume if desired.

Intraperitoneal/Incision Block

Dogs; 2 ml of 2% lidocaine with epinephrine diluted with 2 ml of 0.9% sodium chloride (4 ml total per 4.5 kg of body weight) or 2.0 ml of 0.5% bupivacaine diluted with 2.0 ml of 0.9% sodium chloride (4 ml total per 4.5 kg of body weight).

Complications and Contraindications

♥ Pneumothorax, inadvertent pulmonary trauma during catheter placement, and infection.

✓ Severe peritonitis may cause additional systemic uptake of local anesthetic.

Technical Skill

✓ Positioning of chest tube or catheter requires moderate skill. The remainder of the procedure requires minimal skill.

◉ See CD for demonstration of Interpleural Analgesia/Anesthesia technique (Video 3-10).

Intravenous Constant Rate Infusion

Technique

Intravenous constant rate infusions begin with an intravenous loading dose of the same analgesic to be infused. The technique requires the placement of an indwelling intravenous catheter. The infusion rate can be calculated using several different methods but a method known as dimensional analysis is more intuitive and provides insight into the cause of mistakes in calculation. If analgesic drugs are to be administered with maintenance fluids, the length of infusion will be determined by the volume of maintenance fluid in the bag and rate of fluid administration.

✓ An equivalent volume of fluid should be removed from the IV fluid bag before the drug is added if the exact final concentration calculated is desired. In this example, 20.0 ml of maintenance fluid would be removed and replaced with 20.0 ml of fentanyl (50 mcg/ml) (Table 3-1).

Table 3-1
Example of analgesic drug constant rate infusion calculation by the dimensional analysis method

A 10 kg dog receives 60 ml/kg/day as its maintenance fluid rate. You want to administer fentanyl at 5 mcg/kg/hr.

1. Determine the maintenance fluid administration rate
   Maintenance fluid rate (ml/hr) = (60 ml/kg/day x 10 kg) ÷ 24hr = 25 ml/hr

2. Determine how long the bag of fluids will last (assume a 500 ml bag)
   Duration of maintenance fluid infusion (hr) = 500 ml ÷ 25 ml/hr = 20.0 hrs

3. Determine the amount of analgesic drug to add to the bag of fluids.
   Fentanyl dose (mcg) = 5 mcg/kg/hr of fentanyl x 10 kg x 20.0hr = 1000 mcg

4. Determine the volume of analgesic drug to add to the bag of IV fluid
   (assume the concentration of fentanyl is 50 mcg/ml)
   Fentanyl volume (ml) = 1000 mcg ÷ 50 mcg/ml of fentanyl = 20.0 mls

✔ If the analgesic drug delivery rate is to be changed, you should be careful not to exceed safe rates of maintenance fluid administration. It helps to mix one bag of fluids with the maximum desired concentration of analgesic drug added, and then dilute it to a lower concentration by piggybacking it onto a second unspiked bag of maintenance fluid. By adjusting the rate of the two bags it is possible to adjust the analgesic dose without overhydrating the patient.

Materials Needed

IV fluid bag and administration set
IV catheter

✔ An automated fluid pump or syringe pump may facilitate fluid administration but these are not mandatory if drug administration is closely monitored.

Drugs and Dosages

Morphine (15 mg/ml):
Dogs; loading dose 0.2-0.5 mg/kg, then 0.05-0.3 mg/kg/hr CRI.
Cats; loading dose 0.05-0.1 mg/kg, then 0.025-0.2 mg/kg/hr CRI.

Fentanyl (50 mcg/ml):
Dog; loading dose 2.0-10.0 mcg/kg, then 2-10 mcg/kg/hr CRI.
Cats; loading dose 1.0-5.0 mcg/kg, then 1-5 mcg/kg/hr CRI.

Ketamine (100 mg/ml):
Dogs; loading dose 0.5-2.0 mg/kg, then 0.1-0.5 mg/kg/hr CRI.

Complications and Contraindications

✓ The most common complications are poor analgesia, mild dysphoria, and occasionally CNS depression.

♥ The patient should be assessed periodically for intensity of pain and the dose adjusted to improve analgesia if necessary.

✓ The co-administration of medetomidine or ketamine with opioids, or the intermittent administration of an adjuvant drug such as acepromazine will decrease dysphoria. Reducing the infusion rate usually helps to reduce the incidence of opioid dysphoria and excessive CNS depression.

✓ If done correctly, CRI of analgesic drugs may be the safest route of administration since rapid control of drug delivery is achievable and allows dosing to effect.

Technical Skill

✓ This procedure requires minimal skill.

♥ The patient will require more intensive supervision during the infusion period.

Transdermal Opioid Delivery

Technique

Typical locations for patch placement are on the dorsum of the neck or back for dogs and on the lateral thorax for cats. Some veterinarians have had success in placing patches on the limbs of dogs and cats covered by a padded secure bandage. Location may vary but the patch should be in a place not affected by heating pads since rates of absorption may be altered by temperature changes (Figure 3-11).

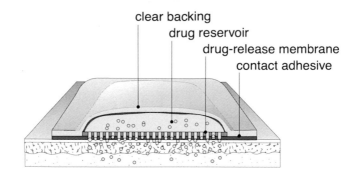

clear backing
drug reservoir
drug-release membrane
contact adhesive

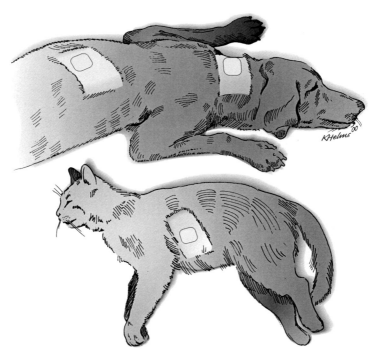

Figure 3-11
Cross-section of the fentanyl patch and placement
locations in dogs and cats

The hair over the desired area is clipped with a surgical clipper blade. The skin should not be shaved since it may disrupt the stratum corneum and alter absorption kinetics. Water should be used to clean the skin before patch application. Alcohol and detergent containing soaps should not be used since they will alter epidermal lipids and absorption. The occlusive backing is then peeled off the patch and it is pressed onto the skin. Cover the patch with an adhesive bandage to improve skin-patch contact and reduce the likelihood of patch loss. There is a lag time ranging from 6 to 24 hours before analgesic effects will be observed. During this period supplemental opioids should be administered if the patient appears to be in pain. Drug absorption from fentanyl patches may vary considerably from patient to patient so the adequacy of analgesia should be assessed frequently and additional analgesics administered as needed.

Materials Needed

Fentanyl transdermal patch (Duragesic®)

Drugs and Dosages

Dogs:
> 10 kg - 25 mcg/hr patch
> 10-20 kg - 50 mcg/hr patch
> 20-30 kg - 75 mcg/hr patch
> >30 kg - 100 mcg/hr patch

Cats:
> 25 mcg/hr patch

✓ For smaller cats, use only one-half of the surface by leaving the occlusive backing over half of the patch.

Complications and Contraindications

✓ Patch application does not insure analgesia.

♥ Analgesic drugs should be administered during the lag time following application of the patch.

💣 Accidental or intentional fentanyl exposure to children or adults should be considered when deciding if the transdermal patch is appropriate or is to be dispensed as a take-home medication.

Technical Skill

✓ This procedure requires minimal skill.

⊙ See CD for demonstration of Transdermal Opioid Delivery technique (Video 3-11).

Adjunctive Analgesic Techniques

Veterinarians have an increasing variety of nonpharmacologic options available for the prevention and treatment of both acute and chronic pain. When possible, early (preemptive) use of non-pharmacologic analgesic techniques is preferred and, similar to analgesic drug administration, improves efficacy of therapy. Alternative analgesic therapies should undergo rigorous clinical testing to validate their role in the future of pain management.

✔ The use of acupuncture needles, moxibustion, injections, lasers, and magnets may constitute a surgical procedure under state veterinary practice acts and should only be performed by a licensed veterinarian who has completed an appropriate educational program on their use.

✔ The AVMA has published proposed guidelines for complementary, alternative, and integrative medicine which state claims for safety and effectiveness should ultimately be proven by scientific methods. Ineffective or unsafe practices should be discarded.

Rehabilitation Therapy

Rehabilitation incorporates physical or mechanical agents such as light, heat, cold, water, electricity, massage, and exercise in the treatment of pain and dysfunction associated with many orthopedic, neurologic, oncologic, and medical conditions. There are six therapeutic modalities used to decrease pain, reduce inflammation, and stimulate normal healing responses in the rehabilitation patient: local hypo- and hyperthermia, massage, therapeutic exercise, hydrotherapy, ultrasound, and electrical stimulation. The incorporation of rehabilitation therapy in the treatment of orthopedic diseases and chronic pain syndromes has proven an effective approach in some canine patients unresponsive to traditional pain management drugs and techniques.

Iontophoretic Application of Local Anesthetics

Lidocaine can be applied topically under an occlusive patch or administered iontophoretically using bipolar electrodes connected to a DC battery system to provide current. In burn-related pain, effective analgesia can be achieved in as little as 5 to 10 minutes using this technique. Numby Stuff® is a commercially available ionotophoretic system producing cutaneous anesthesia up to 10 mm in depth following a 10 min application. Each application device delivers 1 mL of 2% lidocaine with epinephrine to the site. The skin immediately blanches and results in a tingling sensation. At this time veterinary application is minimal.

Acupuncture

Acupuncture has been shown to be effective in controlling acute and chronic pain although its mechanism of action is not yet completely understood. Its interaction with afferent pain and proprioceptive sensory nerves provokes local, spinal, and centrally-mediated control mechanisms. Intact nerves, blood, and lymphatic vessels are required to initiate and sustain the reaction. Acupoints are locations that correspond to known neural networks and are usually close to major nerves. Stimulation of points producing the most intense analgesia typically overlie major nerves. Several theories of the mechanism of action have been suggested, and the effect in any given patient is likely the result of one, several, or all of these. Suggested theories include the neural gate theory mediated by A-delta and A-beta fibers; the neural opiate theory mediated by endorphin release; catecholamines and serotonin inhibitory effects within the spinal cord; the hormonal opiate theory mediated by the release of hormonal factors from the pituitary including substance P, histamine, growth hormone, prolactin, oxytocin and others; the autonomic nervous system interaction theory mediated by A-beta fiber stimulation and vasodilation which counteracts A-delta fiber vasoconstriction and cramping and possibly sympathetically maintained pain.

TENS and TAES

Transcutaneous electrical nerve stimulation (TENS) generates antinociceptive responses secondary to activation of A-beta fibers by cutaneous application of electrical current. It has been used in the treatment of virtually all types of pain in human patients, but seems to be most effective in chronic neuropathic and degenerative arthritic pain. Recently, a new mode of TENS therapy, transcutaneous acupoint electrical stimulation (TAES), which provides intermittent stimulation to acupoints with alternating low-and high-frequency electrical current, has been introduced into clinical practice. Although TAES may not provide sufficient pain relief as a sole modality, it can be useful as an adjuvant to patient controlled analgesia in the management of acute postoperative pain.

PENS

The conceptual basis for percutaneous electrical nerve stimulation (PENS) is related to both transcutaneous electrical nerve stimulation (TENS) and electroacupuncture. The use of PENS has the advantage of allowing you to bypass the resistance of the cutaneous barrier and deliver the electrical stimulus in closer proximity to the nerve endings located in the soft tissue, muscle, and periosteum of the involved dermatomes. Electrical stimulation of the nerve endings located in the periosteum appears to be an important factor in achieving analgesia in patients with bone cancer.

Magnetic Field Induction

Magnetic field induction involves establishing a pulsed magnetic field across the tissue of interest. Though the potential mechanism of action is poorly understood, there are anecdotal reports of its efficacy in managing a variety of clinical pain syndromes in humans.

Neurolytic Techniques

Neurolytic techniques are commonly used in the treatment of intractable malignant cancer pain. Such techniques involve the chemical (alcohol, phenol, aminoglycoside) or physical (cryotherapy, laser therapy, radiation therapy) destruction of a nerve to create a permanent interruption of neural transmission.

Palliative Radiation Therapy

Palliative radiation therapy can reduce or eliminate pain associated with some tumors, such as osteosarcoma. The goal of palliative radiotherapy is to alleviate pain, not to prolong survival or eradicate the tumor. A large dose of radiation per fraction is used and the treatment course is usually one dose per week for three or four weeks. Response to treatment occurs between one and 60 days after initiation of treatment. The duration of response to palliative radiation therapy varies from a few weeks to several months. If relapses occur, the animal may be re-treated.

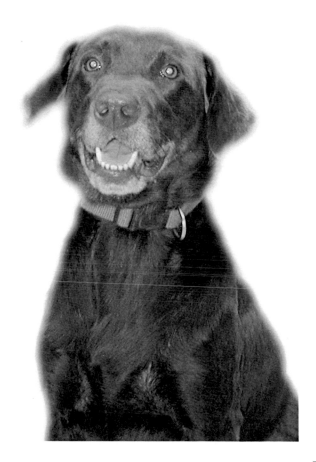

Section 4

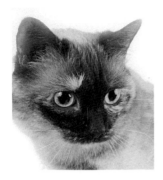

Pain Management for Specific Conditions and Procedures

Initial Pain Management of the Trauma Patient

General Considerations

♥ A thorough physical examination, including a neurological examination, should be performed before any analgesic is administered. Special attention should be given to the cardiovascular, respiratory, and neurological systems. If the patient appears stable then the level of required analgesia can be determined.

✔ If diagnostic procedures are planned, such as a radiographic or ultrasound examination, analgesic or sedative analgesic combinations may facilitate positioning and reduce stress and anxiety.

✔ Take care not to overmedicate the patient which could lead to impaired organ system function and potential worsening of patient condition.

✔ Initial administration of opioids will often prove satisfactory for most types of acute pain. The opioid selected will depend on the severity of trauma and perceived requirements for analgesics.

♥ NSAIDs should be administered cautiously during periods of potential hemorrhage or in anticipation of surgery.

✔ NSAIDs may be less efficacious in the first few hours following trauma than the opioids. NSAID use in any animal with blood loss and the potential for low cardiac output should be minimized.

✔ Duration of NSAID use in cats should be limited because of potential toxicity.

💣 If opioids are to be used in patients with suspected intracranial hypertension, respiratory monitoring is required. Possible hypoventilation associated with high doses of μ agonist opioids may worsen intracranial hypertension causing serious neurological impairment.

💣 Alpha2 adrenergic agonists should not be used in patients with a history of hemorrhage which is difficult to control. Hypertension secondary to alpha2 adrenergic agonist-mediated vasoconstriction may worsen hemorrhage.

Recommendations

✓ For severe soft tissue or orthopedic injuries, morphine, oxymorphone, hydromorphone, or buprenorphine may be satisfactory. For less severe injuries, butorphanol may provide adequate short term relief.

✓ Intravenous, intramuscular, subcutaneous, or a continuous rate infusion may be used for drug delivery. A continuous rate infusion will allow rapid titration of the level of analgesia and quick withdrawal of the drug should adverse effects arise.

✓ Intravenous bolus administration is sometimes used to determine the initial analgesic requirement for opioids, with subsequent equivalent doses given by the intramuscular or subcutaneous routes.

✓ Addition of low doses of a sedative/analgesic like medetomidine or a tranquilizer like acepromazine or diazepam may facilitate positioning for diagnostic procedures or calm an anxious patient.

✓ If a fentanyl patch is to be applied, it should be placed as early as possible. Supplemental opioids should be administered for the first 12 to 24 hours. Periodic assessment of analgesic efficacy of the patch should be performed and additional opioids or analgesic drugs given if necessary.

NOTE Refer to Section 2, Tables 2-1, 2-2, 2-3, 2-4, 2-5, and 2-6, for drug dosages and contraindications and Section 3, for applicable techniques in dogs and cats.

⊙ See CD for Transdermal Opioid Delivery (Video 3-11), various Regional Nerve Blocks, and Infiltrative Blocks (Video 3-7).

Head Trauma
Anticipated Degree of Pain
Mild to Severe

✓ The level of pain associated with head trauma may be difficult to assess due to changes in normal behavior and mentation.

♥ A thorough physical examination including a neurological examination should be performed before any pharmacologic alteration of CNS activity occurs. Vital signs and neurological status should be closely monitored and appropriate supportive therapy initiated if necessary.

Preemptive Analgesic Medications

✓ The traumatic nature of these injuries precludes the use of preemptive analgesics.

Regional Analgesic Techniques

✓ Mandibular and maxillary nerve blocks may be useful for fractures or injuries of the maxilla and mandible.

Postoperative Analgesic Medications

✓ Opioids may be beneficial for severe pain associated with head trauma.

☙ If there is any indication of intracranial hypertension, respiration should be closely monitored before and after high doses of opioids or other drugs which may affect respiration are administered. **Remember that minute ventilation is the important parameter to monitor.** Changes in respiratory rate or tidal volume alone are not enough to gauge respiratory depression. Use of arterial blood gas monitoring or capnometry will more accurately monitor changes in ventilation. Hypercapnea, regardless of the cause, will tend to increase cerebral blood flow and potentiate intracranial hypertension. Patients with head trauma may also be at risk for seizure activity following injury.

✓ Administration of drugs that are known to precipitate seizure activity are contraindicated.

Dispensable Analgesic Medications

✓ NSAIDs and NSAID/opioid combinations have been used as post head-trauma analgesics. Oral opioid agonists may be useful in some difficult cases as the primary analgesic. Presently there are no available NSAID/opioid combination products available for safe use in cats.

💣✳ If signs of intracranial hemorrhage are present, NSAIDs are contraindicated.

Example Protocol

Dog: Premedication with atropine (0.044 mg/kg)+hydromorphone (0.2 mg/kg) given intramuscularly 20 minutes before induction with thiopental or propofol. Anesthetic maintenance is accomplished with isoflurane (also preferred in patients with a history of thoracic trauma or cardiac arrhythmias). Post-operative continuous rate infusions of opioids can be used in patients with severe pain. In patients with signs of intracranial hypertension it is important to monitor ventilation.

NOTE Refer to Section 2, Tables 2-1, 2-2, 2-4, 2-7, 2-8, and 2-9, for drug dosages and Section 3, for applicable techniques for dogs and cats.

⊙ See CD for demonstration of Dental Nerve Blocks (Video 3-6).

Acute Pancreatitis
Anticipated Degree of Pain

Moderate to Severe

✓ Acute pancreatitis is usually associated with visceral pain.

Preemptive Analgesic Medications

✓ The acute onset of this disease precludes the preemptive use of analgesics.

Regional Analgesic Technique

✓ Epidural administration of opioids or alpha$_2$ adrenergic agonists have been used to treat pain associated with pancreatitis or other types of abdominal lesions. Lumbosacral epidural injection of opioids with low lipophilicity such as morphine should provide some relief.

Lipophilic opioids such as fentanyl or buprenorphine require delivery closer to the site of afferent input into the spinal cord and may be delivered by an epidural catheter. The catheter tip should be advanced to the thoracolumbar area of the spine. Epidural catheter placement should be done under heavy sedation or anesthesia to prevent patient movement when performing this technique.

✓ Interpleural local anesthetic administration may also provide relief for pancreatitis pain. Nerves innervating the cranial abdomen enter the spinal cord in the caudal thoracic region. Interpleural catheter placement may be beneficial if the need for repeated local anesthetic administration is anticipated.

Postoperative Analgesic Medications

✓ Acute pancreatitis most often does not require surgical correction.

Dispensable Analgesic Medication

✓ Vomiting and gastrointestinal dysfunction which often occur with pancreatitis will make oral administration of analgesic drugs difficult in some patients.

✓ Oral medications may be contraindicated if the patient is still NPO as part of the treatment plan.

✓ Fentanyl patches have been popular for treatment of pancreatitis-associated pain. Supplemental opioids should be given until the level of analgesia from the fentanyl patch appears satisfactory. Also, the adequacy of analgesia should be periodically assessed to assure the patient is comfortable.

Example Protocol

Following diagnosis of acute pancreatitis, the parenteral administration of opioid agonists such as hydromorphone, morphine, and fentanyl provide relief to most patients with severe pain. A fentanyl patch can be applied as soon as possible. Consider placing an epidural catheter or administering local anesthetic into the caudal thoracic space or cranial peritoneal cavity.

✓ Management of acute pancreatic pain in cats can be approached in a similar fashion as described for dogs with the appropriate modification of dosages and techniques.

NOTE Refer to Section 2, Tables 2-1, 2-3, and 2-6, for drug dosages and Section 3 for techniques.

⊙ See CD for demonstration of Epidural Anesthesia (Video 3-1), Epidural Catheter Placement (Video 3-2), Interpleural analgesia (Video 3-10) and Transdermal Opioid Delivery (Video 3-11) techniques.

Canine Procedures
Dental Cleaning with Extractions
Anticipated Degree of Pain
Mild to Moderate

The degree of pain depends on the level of preexisting dental disease and location and number of teeth extracted.

Preemptive Analgesic Medications

✓ Oral or injectable NSAIDs and opioids are the analgesics most commonly used. One or two doses are typically given before the procedure.

✓ Newer NSAIDs such as carprofen, deracoxib or meloxicam can be used perioperatively because of their minimal effects on hemostasis.

✓ Premedication with analgesic drugs such as opioids and low doses of alpha$_2$ adrenergic agonists may reduce overall postoperative analgesic requirements.

Regional Analgesic Techniques

✓ Mandibular, maxillary, and infra-orbital nerve blocks may be used before extraction to reduce postoperative pain.

✎※ Patients may react to a loss of sensation to the lips or tongue by chewing which can result in self-mutilation. The probability of self-mutilation may be greater when bilateral blocks desensitize an entire region of the mouth.

Postoperative Analgesic Medications

✓ There is evidence from human experience that NSAIDs alone or in combination with codeine or other opioids provide excellent analgesia without causing excessive sedation or side effects.

✓ For extreme procedures, such as whole mouth extractions or multiple molar extractions, several doses of a full μ agonist like morphine or hydromorphone may be required for patient comfort in addition to daily NSAID administration.

Dispensable Analgesic Medications

✓ Oral NSAIDs are the most widely recommended dispensable analgesic drugs for short-term treatment of pain associated with canine dental procedures. Additional take home analgesia may be provided with butorphanol tablets alone or in combination with NSAIDs.

Example Protocol

Premedication with medetomidine (8.0 mcg/kg) + butorphanol (0.2 mg/kg) + atropine (0.044 mg/kg) given intramuscularly 20 minutes before induction with either thiopental, propofol, or ketamine given "to effect" intravenously. Maintain anesthesia with halothane or isoflurane. Appropriate regional nerve blocks may be performed to reduce the amount of postoperative pain. Postoperative analgesia can be provided with a number of oral NSAIDs such as carprofen and an opioid, if necessary.

✓ Management of dental pain in cats can be approached in a similar fashion as described for dogs with the appropriate modification of dosages and techniques. Twice or three times a day transmucosal buprenorphine administration is a good alternative to butorphanol oral administration in cats. NSAIDs should be used at reduced doses from those recommended for dogs. Acetaminophen is toxic to cats.

NOTE Refer to Section 2, Figure 2-1, Tables 2-1, 2-2, 2-3, 2-4, 2-7, 2-8, and 2-9 for drug dosages and Section 3 for applicable techniques.

◉ See CD for demonstration of Mandibular, Maxillary, and Infraorbital Nerve Block techniques (Video 3-6).

Ovariohysterectomy
Anticipated Degree of Pain
Mild to Moderate

The intensity of pain expressed by any particular patient is a function of surgical technique and the animal's pain tolerance.

Preemptive Analgesic Medications

✓ When no contraindications are present, oral or injectable NSAIDs may be effective preemptive analgesics. Carprofen is approved for perioperative pain control for soft tissue surgery in dogs.

✓ Premedication with alpha$_2$ adrenergic agonists, opioids, and other analgesic drugs often reduce anesthetic and postoperative analgesic requirements.

Regional Analgesic Techniques

✓ Regional nerve blocks are not typically performed for routine abdominal surgery.

✓ Intraperitoneal local anesthetics have been advocated for some laparoscopic and laparotomy procedures.

✓ Infiltration of the incision site with local anesthetics provides some postoperative analgesia.

Postoperative Analgesic Medications

✓ Injectable NSAIDs, opioids, and analgesic adjuvant drugs such as alpha$_2$ adrenergic agonists or other sedatives can be used to reduce the pain and stress experienced by some patients following OHE surgery. Typically, opioids prove efficacious immediately following the surgery and NSAIDs are prescribed for longer term pain treatment.

🔥 Animals with bleeding disorders, pregnant animals, or those in estrus may be more prone to bleeding from NSAID mediated platelet inhibition.

Dispensable Analgesic Medications

✓ Oral NSAIDs or a combination of acetaminophen with codeine are the most widely recommended dispensable analgesic drugs for short-term treatment of postoperative pain following canine OHE. Additional dispensable medications include butorphanol tablets given alone or in combination with NSAIDs. In most patients 3-4 days of analgesic therapy is sufficient.

Example Protocol

Premedication with injectable carprofen (2-4 mg/kg, SC) followed by medetomidine (8.0 mcg/kg) + butorphanol (0.2 mg/kg) + atropine (0.044 mg/kg) given intramuscularly. Induction of anesthesia can be achieved 20 minutes later with either thiopental, propofol, or ketamine given "to effect" intravenously. Maintain anesthesia with halothane or isoflurane. Postoperative analgesia can be provided by an injectable NSAID such as carprofen if not given preemptively and either butorphanol or buprenorphine, if necessary.

♠* If immediate pain relief is required, intravenous opioids will provide relief more rapidly than an NSAID and should be given first.

NOTE Refer to Section 2, Figure 2-1, Tables 2-1, 2-2, 2-3, 2-4, 2-5, 2-6, 2-7, 2-8, and 2-9, for drug dosages and Section 3 for applicable techniques.

◉ See CD for demonstration of Infiltrative Block technique (Video 3-7).

Castration

Anticipated Degree of Pain

Mild to Moderate

♥ The level of pain experienced by any particular patient is a function of surgical technique and the animal's pain tolerance. Analgesics should not be withheld because the practitioner believes the level of pain displayed by the patient is less than expected.

Preemptive Analgesic Medications

✓ Oral or injectable NSAIDs may be effective preemptive analgesics when given before or during surgery.

✓ Premedication with alpha₂ adrenergic agonists, opioids, and other analgesic drugs may reduce anesthetic and postoperative analgesic requirements.

Regional Analgesic Technique

✓ Infiltration of the spermatic cord before ligation and transection may decrease the sympathetic nervous system response and pain associated with ligature application while reducing anesthetic requirements.

Postoperative Analgesic Medications

✓ Injectable NSAIDs, opioids, and analgesic adjuvant drugs such as alpha₂ adrenergic agonists can be used to reduce pain and stress experienced by some patients following castration.

✔ Typically, opioids prove efficacious immediately following the surgery and NSAIDs may be prescribed for longer term treatment.

✔ Animals with bleeding disorders may be more prone to scrotal bleeding due to platelet inhibition induced by some NSAIDs.

Dispensable Analgesic Medications

✔ Oral NSAIDs or butorphanol tablets are the most widely recommended dispensable analgesic drugs for short-term treatment of postoperative pain associated with canine castration. Additional analgesia may be provided by combining butorphanol tablets with an NSAID such as carprofen.

Example Protocol

Injectable carprofen (2-4 mg/kg, SC) can be followed by premedication with acepromazine (0.05 mg/kg) + hydromorphone (0.1 mg/kg) or butorphanol (0.2 mg/kg) + atropine (0.044 mg/kg) given intramuscularly 20 minutes before induction with either thiopental, propofol, or ketamine given "to effect" intravenously. Maintain anesthesia with halothane or isoflurane. Postoperative analgesia can be provided with an NSAID if not given preemptively and additional opioid if necessary.

NOTE Refer to Section 2, Figure 2-1, Tables 2-1, 2-2, 2-3, 2-4, 2-5, 2-7, 2-8, and 2-9 for drug dosages and Section 3 for applicable techniques.

⊙ See CD for demonstration of Infiltrative Block technique (Video 3-7).

Exploratory Laparotomy/ Cystotomy

Anticipated Degree of Pain

Mild to Severe

Some canine patients will experience severe pain and distress following laparotomy or cystostomy while others appear to experience almost none.

♥ The outward display of pain and stress should not be a requirement for analgesic administration. Some of the difference in response may be related to animal behavior and conditioning. Stoic animals will often remain untreated for their pain because they do not "ask for it." It is generally accepted that all patients should be treated if the possibility of pain exists and the animal will not be adversely affected by analgesic administration.

✓ Intense pain and stress, whether displayed or quietly tolerated, can reduce immune function, delay wound healing, and potentially lead to chronic painful conditions which are difficult to treat.

Preemptive Analgesic Medications

✓ Abdominal exploration is performed for numerous conditions such as removal of splenic tumors, cystotomy, and foreign body removal. Choice of preemptive analgesic drugs should be made with consideration given to other cardiovascular, respiratory, or physiological disturbances that may be present. For example, NSAID administration may be contraindicated if gastrointestinal or renal pathology has been present or if the risk for low blood pressure exists prior to or during anesthesia and surgery.

✓ Opioids (hydromorphone, morphine, or buprenorphine) are generally preferred for preemptive analgesic administration due to their favorable safety profile and excellent analgesic properties in dogs.

✓ One caveat is the administration of analgesic drugs that can cause vomiting (such as opioids and alpha$_2$ adrenergic agonists) to animals with gastrointestinal disease and gastric or intestinal foreign body.

♥ Generalities about appropriate drug selection cannot be made for a laparotomy. Specific drug selection should be based on specific patient pathophysiology at the time of surgery.

Regional Analgesic Techniques

✓ The use of epidural analgesia/anesthesia is not common due to the increased cost, time, and potential for complications. Never the less, an epidural block may be useful for some types of surgery which require profound muscle relaxation or when straining must be prevented postoperatively.

✓ Epidural morphine administration, although long lasting in effect, may be contraindicated following cystotomy because of the increased incidence of urine retention and potential for increased pressure on the cystotomy suture line. Similar concerns extend to the use of transdermal fentanyl patches which may be associated impaired urinary bladder voiding in some patients.

✔ Infiltration of the incision site with local anesthetic provides immediate postoperative analgesia.

Postoperative Analgesic Medications

✔ Injectable NSAIDs, opioids, and analgesic adjuvant drugs such as alpha$_2$ adrenergic agonists and other sedatives can be used to reduce the pain and stress experienced by some patients following abdominal surgery. Fentanyl (2-5 mcg/kg/h) given as a continuous rate intravenous infusion is efficacious immediately following surgery. NSAIDs may be prescribed for longer term treatment.

💣 Animals with a history of gastrointestinal bleeding or coagulopathies may be more prone to hemorrhage due to inhibition of prostaglandin synthesis and platelet function. NSAIDs are contraindicated in these patients.

✔ A growing body of evidence indicates that the continuous intravenous infusion of lidocaine (without epinephrine) during and after anesthesia may improve bowel function in patients undergoing abdominal surgery. Intravenous lidocaine infusion may also reduce overall analgesic drug requirement and the incidence of ventricular arrhythmias. The combination of lidocaine, ketamine, and full opioid agonist such as morphine or hydromorphone when administered in low doses via CRI may be beneficial in preventing central hypersensitization and a resultant chronic pain state.

Dispensable Analgesic Medications

✔ Oral NSAIDs or acetaminophen with codeine or oxycodone are good dispensable analgesic drugs for pain associated with canine abdominal surgery unrelated to gastrointestinal or renal pathology. Minimal analgesia may be provided with butorphanol tablets alone.

Example Protocol

✔ Opioids administered preemptively are typically included in the majority of anesthetic plans. Induction with any of the intravenous induction agents is appropriate unless a specific contraindication exists. Maintenance is accomplished with isoflurane or halothane in oxygen and post-operative pain control with opioids.

✔ Nonpharmacologic techniques such as hot packing may provide additional relief from discomfort associated with swelling and inflammation.

✓ Management of abdominal surgical pain in cats can be approached in a similar fashion with the appropriate species modification of dosages and techniques.

NOTE Refer to Section 2, Figure 2-1, Tables 2-1, 2-2, 2-3, 2-4, 2-5, 2-6, 2-7, 2-8, and 2-9 for drug dosages and Section 3 for applicable techniques.

⊙ See CD for demonstration of Epidural Analgesia (Video 3-1) and Infiltrative Block (Video 3-7).

Forelimb Amputation/Fracture

Anticipated Degree of Pain

Moderate to severe

✓ Depends upon the degree and site of fracture and participation in weight bearing.

Preemptive Analgesic Medications

✓ Preemptive analgesia is typically not an option in cases of traumatic or pathologic fractures.

✓ Early administration of analgesic drugs upon presentation may help reduce the occurrence of secondary changes in neuroprocessing (allodynia and hyperalgesia).

✓ Opioids are probably most efficacious against fracture pain. Addition of NSAIDs or alpha$_2$ adrenergic agonists with the opioid will often enhance analgesia, prolong duration of effect, and improve analgesic response in difficult cases.

✒* Patients with a history of fracture secondary to trauma should be thoroughly examined for signs of thoracic, abdominal, or cranial trauma.

Regional Analgesic Techniques

✓ Brachial plexus nerve block may be effective for fractures distal to the shoulder.

✓ The proximal radial/median/ulnar nerve block is efficacious for relieving discomfort due to fractures distal to the elbow.

✓ Local infiltrative ring blocks have been used for temporary relief of pain associated with surgery or trauma of the distal forelimb.

✓ Epidural administration of morphine via lumbosacral puncture may be effective as far forward as the forelimb.

💣※ Remember that cranial migration of local anesthetics to the cranial thoracic and/or cervical spinal cord can be associated with respiratory and sympathetic dysfunction. Large doses of local anesthetics are *not* recommended for epidural administration to extend analgesia cranial to the thoracolumbar junction.

✓ In patients non-responsive to pain medications or when contraindications to traditional analgesic drug therapy are present, electroacupuncture may prove beneficial in some cases.

✓ Forelimb amputation pain may be treated with the placement of a sterile fenestrated catheter buried within the surgical incision site connected to an elastomeric delivery system (Pain Buster®) designed to deliver local anesthetic at a constant rate (0.5-5.0 ml/h for up to 5 days).

Postoperative Analgesic Medications

✓ Injectable opioid administration is probably the most efficacious method of pain relief for the immediate postinjury or postsurgical period. Adjuvant agents will provide additional analgesia and sedation in patients with pain that is difficult to control.

✓ When combined with opioids, microdose ketamine administration (0.5 mg/kg followed by 2-10 mcg/kg/min CRI for the first day or 2 postoperatively) may prove beneficial.

✓ Fentanyl patches can be efficacious and provide a reasonable length of analgesia but supplemental opioids will be required for the first 12 to 24 hours until adequate analgesia is achieved. Patients should be examined periodically and given additional analgesics if they appear uncomfortable following fentanyl patch application.

Dispensable Analgesic Medications

✓ Oral NSAIDs and NSAID/opioid combinations can be used as short term dispensable analgesics when hemostasis is not a concern.

✓ Some practitioners feel comfortable dispensing fentanyl patches for home use.

✓ Acetaminophen and codeine or oxycodone may be an excellent NSAID/opioid combination for 2 to 3 days of postoperative pain control following fracture repair in canine patients.

✓ Butorphanol tablets improve analgesia when combined with NSAID administration.

✓ For the first few days following fracture repair or forelimb amputation in a cat, buprenorphine (0.01-0.02 mg/kg) can be administered every 8 hours transmucosally along with oral meloxicam (0.1 mg/kg initial dose followed by 0.025 mg/kg for subsequent doses).

Example Protocol

Premedication with medetomidine (8.0 mcg/kg) + atropine (0.044 mg/kg) + morphine (0.5 mg/kg) given intramuscularly 20 minutes before induction with either thiopental, propofol, or ketamine given "to effect" intravenously. Maintain anesthesia with halothane or isoflurane (isoflurane is preferred with a history of thoracic trauma or cardiac arrhythmias). A brachial plexus block can be performed before surgery. Intra- and postoperative continuous rate infusions of opioids can be used with severe injuries.

✓ Management of fracture pain in cats can be approached in a similar fashion as described for dogs with the appropriate modification of dosages and techniques.

NOTE Refer to Section 2, Tables 2-1, 2-2, 2-3, 2-4, 2-5, 2-6, 2-7, 2-8, and 2-9 for drug dosages and Section 3 for applicable techniques.

⊙ See CD for demonstration of Brachial Plexus Nerve Block (Video 3-3), Proximal Radial/Ulnar/Median Nerve Blocks (Video 3-4), Transdermal Opioid Delivery (Video 3-11), and Epidural Block (Video 3-1).

Thoracotomy
Anticipated Degree of Pain
Moderate to Severe

✓ Median sternotomy is considered a more painful procedure by some, but any thoracotomy may cause signs of respiratory impairment secondary to pain of breathing.

Preemptive Analgesic Medications

✓ Most thoracotomies are scheduled, so that the preemptive administration of analgesic drugs such as opioids, alpha$_2$ adrenergic agonists, and NSAIDs are an option.

♥ Selection of an appropriate preemptive analgesic is based on understanding the disease process underlying the need for surgery.

Regional Analgesic Techniques

✓ Intercostal nerve blocks or interpleural analgesic administration with local anesthetics and/or epidural administration of opioids can be used to provide regional analgesia prior to or following thoracotomy.

✓ Interpleural analgesic administration may be preferable if a chest tube is in place. Repeat administration of interpleural local anesthetics can occur for as long as the chest tube is in position.

✓ Epidural administration should be limited to opioids or adjuvant drugs other than local anesthetics. Morphine can be effective when administered at the lumbosacral junction due to its low lipid solubility and diffusibility to the cranial thoracic cord.

✓ Epidural catheter placement at the level of the thorax is an option when long-term administration of analgesics is anticipated.

Postoperative Analgesic Medications

✓ Injectable opioid administration is probably the most efficacious method of pain relief for the immediate postsurgical period.

✓ Fentanyl patches can be efficacious and provide a reasonable length of analgesia but supplemental opioids will be required for the first 12 to 24 hours. Presurgical application is recommended. Patients should be examined periodically and given additional analgesics if they appear uncomfortable after patch application.

✓ Interpleural administration of the long acting local anesthetic bupivacaine is a good method of providing analgesia immediately following thoracotomy.

Dispensable Analgesic Medications

✓ Oral NSAIDs and NSAID/opioid combinations can be effective short term analgesics in dogs.

✓ Opioids (such as butorphanol tablets in dogs, or transmucosal buprenorphine in cats) may enhance analgesia beyond that achieved with NSAID therapy alone.

Example Protocol

Premedication with atropine (0.044 mg/kg) + hydromorphone (0.2 mg/kg) and acepromazine (0.02 mg/kg) given intramuscularly or subcutaneously 20 minutes before induction with either thiopental, propofol, or ketamine given "to effect" intravenously. Anesthetic maintenance is accomplished with isoflurane. Intra- and postoperative continuous rate infusions of opioids can be used in patients with severe pain. Interpleural bupivacaine (1.5 mg/kg) is typically administered through the chest tube following surgery. Thoracotomies are performed for a wide range of underlying conditions and each patient should be evaluated for potential contraindications to any protocol.

✓ Management of thoracic surgical pain in cats can be approached in a similar fashion as described for dogs with the appropriate modification of dosages and techniques.

NOTE Refer to Section 2, Figure 2-1, Tables 2-1, 2-2, 2-5, 2-6, 2-7, 2-8, and 2-9 for drug dosages and Section 3 for applicable techniques.

⊙ See CD for demonstration of Intercostal Nerve Block (Video 3-9), Interpleural Block (Video 3-10), Epidural Anesthesia (Video 3-1), Epidural Catheter Placement (Video 3-2), and Transdermal Opioid Delivery (Video 3-11).

Intervertebral Disc Disease
Anticipated Degree of Pain
Moderate to Severe

✓ Acute intervertebral disk disease (Hansen's type I) affecting hind limb function is typically accompanied by loss of superficial pain and sometimes deep pain. Manipulation of the area posterior to the lesion is usually not associated with severe discomfort. However, surgery is often followed by several days of moderate to severe pain.

✓ Chronic intervertebral disk disease (Hansen's type II) and those types affecting the cervical area are typically accompanied by moderate to severe pain, often with chronic components manifested as allodynia and hyperalgesia. Poor response to NSAIDs and opioids in these patients suggests that a more aggressive or alternative pain management strategy is required.

Preemptive Analgesic Medications

✓ Preemptive analgesia is usually not possible for animals suffering from intervertebral disk disease.

💣* Preoperative use of NSAIDs may cause uncontrollable hemorrhage during surgery. Their use is contraindicated as preemptive medication.

✓ Commonly used analgesic drugs are often less efficacious if a degree of chronic pain has been established.

Regional Analgesic Technique

✓ Local anesthetics are occasionally applied directly to the spinal cord during the final stages of a dorsal laminectomy surgery.

Postoperative Analgesic Medications

✓ Injectable opioid administration is the most efficacious method of pain relief for the immediate postsurgical period. Addition of adjuvant agents (such as low doses of ketamine) may improve analgesia in patients that are unresponsive to opioid therapy.

✓ Fentanyl patches provide a reasonable length of analgesia, but supplemental opioids will be required for the the first 12 to 24 hours. Patients should be examined periodically and given additional analgesics if they appear uncomfortable following patch application.

✓ Patients with a chronic or neuropathic pain component may respond to oral or parenteral administration of low doses of ketamine or tricyclic antidepressants such as amitriptyline or imipramine. Acupuncture or other analgesic techniques may also prove effective (see Section 5).

Dispensable Analgesic Medications

✓ Oral NSAIDs and NSAID/opioid combinations can be used as dispensable analgesics in dogs.

♥ If analgesics are administered as part of medical treatment for intervertebral disk disease, the owner must be informed of the absolute requirement for cage rest and limited physical activity. Analgesics may relieve enough pain that the patient attempts normal activity. Resumption of normal activity may reinjure the cord.

💣* Because an increased incidence of adverse gastrointestinal and/or renal effects occurs when corticosteroids and NSAIDs are coadministered, this practice is contraindicated.

Example Protocol

Premedication with medetomidine (8.0 mcg/kg) + atropine (0.044 mg/kg) + morphine (0.5 mg/kg) given intramuscularly 20 minutes before induction with either thiopental, propofol, or ketamine given "to effect" intravenously. Anesthesia is maintained with a combination of low dose fentanyl and halothane or isoflurane. Mu opioid agonists such as morphine or hydromorphone with or without a tranquilizer are commonly administered following surgery to reduce pain and keep the patient calm.

✓ Management of neurosurgical pain in cats can be approached in a similar fashion as described for dogs with the appropriate modification of dosages and techniques.

NOTE Refer to Section 2, Figure 2-1, Tables 2-1, 2-2, 2-3, 2-5, 2-6, 2-7, 2-8, and 2-9 for drug dosages and Section 3 for applicable techniques.

⊙ See CD for demonstration of Transdermal Opioid Delivery (Video 3-11) technique.

Cruciate Ligament Repair

Anticipated Degree of Pain

Moderate to Severe

✓ Cruciate ligament damage usually results in lameness and discomfort to the patient. Surgical repair of the ligament involving an arthrotomy is usually associated with extreme discomfort immediately following recovery.

Preemptive Analgesic Medications

✓ Preemptive analgesia is not an option in cases of cruciate ligament rupture but analgesics can be administered before surgical correction. Early administration of analgesic drugs may help reduce the occurrence of secondary changes in neuroprocessing (e.g., allodynia and hyperalgesia).

✓ Opioids are probably the most efficacious drugs for moderate to severe acute pain. Addition of NSAIDs or alpha$_2$ adrenergic agonists will often enhance and/or prolong analgesia.

Regional Analgesic Techniques

✓ Epidural administration of local anesthetics, alone or in combination with morphine, provides complete blockade of surgical stimulation if done before surgery. Many patients with epidural local anesthetic/opioid administration do not require additional analgesics for several hours.

✓ Intra-articular administration of bupivacaine and morphine (0.1 mg/kg) can also be quite effective. The volume of local anesthetic and/or morphine should be sufficient to cause slight distension of of the joint capsule.

Postoperative Analgesic Medications

✓ Opioid administration is recommended for patients with severe pain. Adjuvants such as acepromazine may enhance opioid analgesia and sedation in patients with difficult to control pain.

✓ Injectable NSAIDs are useful for controlling pain, inflammation and swelling following cruciate ligament repair. When implementing rehabilitation exercises pain control will improve the attitude and cooperation of the patient.

Dispensable Analgesic Medications

✓ Oral NSAIDs and NSAID/opioid combinations can be used as short term postsurgical analgesics in canine patients. Oral opioids (e.g., butorphanol or morphine tablets) can be helpful in some difficult cases when NSAID therapy alone proves ineffective.

Example Protocol

Premedication with medetomidine (8.0 mcg/kg) + atropine (0.044 mg/kg) + morphine (0.5 mg/kg) given intramuscularly 20 minutes before induction with either thiopental, propofol, or ketamine given "to effect" intravenously. Maintain anesthesia with halothane or isoflurane. After induction, but before surgery, epidural administration of morphine (0.2 mg/kg) q.s. to 1 ml / 4.5 kg with bupivacaine (0.5%) will provide intraoperative analgesia/anesthesia and a less painful recovery. Alternatively, intrarticular administration of bupivacaine (0.5% solution) and morphine (0.1 mg/kg) may be helpful in producing immediate post operative pain control. An NSAID such as carprofen (4 mg/kg) can be administered once daily for several days to weeks following surgery. Effectiveness of rehabilitation therapy is often improved when accompanied by adequate pain control achieved with NSAID administration and/or acupuncture treatments prior to therapy sessions.

✓ Management of pelvic limb surgical pain in cats can be approached in a similar fashion as described for dogs with the appropriate modification of dosages and techniques.

NOTE Refer to Section 2, Figure 2-1, Tables 2-1, 2-2, 2-3, 2-4, 2-5, 2-6, 2-7, 2-8, and 2-9 for drug dosages and Section 3 for applicable techniques.

⊙ See CD for demonstration of Epidural Anesthesia (Video 3-1), and Intra-articular Analgesia (Video 3-5) techniques.

Hind Limb Amputation/Fracture

Anticipated Degree of Pain

Severe

Preemptive Analgesic Medications

✓ Most amputations are performed for irreparable tissue damage or cancer. There is often a component of acute and/or chronic pain present before the animal presents for surgery.

✓ Initial pain therapy following fractures can be achieved with injectable opioids such as morphine, hydromorphone, or fentanyl. Anxiety and stress can be further reduced with co-administration of low doses of tranquilizers such as acepromazine or medetomidine.

✓ True preemptive administration of analgesics before injury is usually not possible, but regional nerve blocks with local anesthetics before surgery may be beneficial by reducing intraoperative anesthetic requirements and preventing development of phantom limb pain.

Regional Analgesic Techniques

✓ Epidural administration of local anesthetics combined with opioids is the preferred analgesic technique.

✓ Patients that display a chronic component of pain may benefit from the addition of ketamine to the epidural injection of local anesthetic and opioid.

✓ In cases requiring intensive therapy, continuous epidural catheters allow for repeated administration of analgesic drugs.

✓ Perineural administration of local anesthetic solutions during the surgical transection of major nerves may also help prevent phantom limb pain. Pain originating from tissue disruption proximal to the site of nerve ligation will not be inhibited.

Postoperative Analgesic Medications

✓ Injectable opioid administration is probably the most efficacious method of pain relief for the immediate postsurgical period. Adding adjuvant agents such as ketamine, acepromazine, or gabapentin will often improve analgesia and sedation.

✓ If there are no contraindications to their use, NSAIDs are useful for less severe pain and pain associated with inflammation and swelling.

✓ Administration of opioids, alpha$_2$ adrenergic agonists, and local anesthetics via an indwelling epidural catheter may be required for refractory cases. A continuous intravenous infusion of a μ receptor opioid agonist such as morphine (0.1 mg/kg/h) or fentanyl (3-10 mcg/kg/h) is effective in the immediate postoperative period.

✓ The use of a continuous delivery of local anesthetic via a fenestrated catheter system (Pain Buster® Soaker) inserted under a large incision can provide pain relief for several days following amputation of the rear limb.

Dispensable Analgesic Medications

✓ Oral NSAIDs and NSAID/opioid combinations can be used as short term post-surgical analgesics in canine patients. For example, sustained release oral morphine (1 mg/kg, PO BID) or tramadol (2-10 mg/kg, PO BID or TID) along with once a day NSAID administration (4 mg/kg carprofen, PO) may provide good pain control for several days following surgery.

Example Protocol

Premedication with medetomidine (8.0 mcg/kg) + atropine (0.044 mg/kg) + morphine (0.5 mg/kg) given intramuscularly 20 minutes before induction with either ketamine, thiopental, or propofol given "to effect" intravenously. Anesthetic maintenance is accomplished with halothane or isoflurane. After induction, but before surgery, epidural administration of morphine (0.1-0.2 mg/kg) q.s. to 1 ml / 4.5kg with bupivacaine (0.5%) will help provide intraoperative analgesia/anesthesia and smooth recovery. If an epidural catheter has been inserted for repeated administration, the dose of bupivacaine can be decreased to 0.1 mg/kg on subsequent administrations to minimize motor nerve blockade.

✓ Management of hind limb amputation pain in cats can be approached in a similar fashion as described for dogs with the appropriate modification of dosages and techniques.

NOTE Refer to Section 2, Figure 2-1, Tables 2-1, 2-2, 2-3, 2-4, 2-5, 2-6, 2-7, 2-8, and 2-9 for drug dosages and Section 3 for applicable techniques.

◉ See CD for demonstration of Intravenous Regional Anesthesia (Video 3-8), Epidural Anesthesia (Video 3-1), Epidural Catheter Placement (Video 3-2), and Transdermal Opioid Delivery (Video 3-11) techniques.

Degloving Injury
Anticipated Degree of Pain
Mild to Severe

✓ The amount of tissue injury may or may not reflect the degree of pain experienced by the patient. If ligament or bone damage has also occurred pain may be more intense.

✓ The chronic nature of degloving injuries may predispose this subpopulation of trauma patients to altered central nervous system processing. Early administration of analgesic adjuvant agents such as ketamine (NMDA antagonist) may be warranted to help reduce the development of peripheral and central hypersensitization.

Preemptive Analgesic Medications

✓ Preemptive analgesia is usually not possible due to the traumatic nature of these injuries.

✓ Aggressive treatment with opioid and opioid combinations (e.g., with NMDA antagonists such as ketamine), with the aim of preventing changes in pain processing, may be helpful.

Regional Analgesic Techniques

✓ For pelvic limb degloving injuries, the epidural administration of opioids, local anesthetics, and adjuvant drugs such as ketamine may prove helpful. Epidural administration of morphine but not local anesthetics can be tried for forelimb degloving injuries.

✓ Specific regional nerve block techniques may also be beneficial for short term treatment of pain (e.g., brachial plexus block for forelimb degloving injury).

Postoperative Analgesic Medications

✓ Injectable opioid administration is probably the most efficacious method of pain relief in patients with severe pain.

✓ Administration of opioids, and local anesthetics via an indwelling epidural catheter may be required for refractory cases.

✓ An intravenous continuous rate infusion of fentanyl or morphine can be used in the immediate postoperative period.

Dispensable Analgesic Medications

✓ Oral NSAIDs and NSAID/opioid combinations are recommended for post-trauma analgesic administration in dogs.

✓ In cats, an oral opioid such as buprenorphine (0.01-0.02 mg/kg, transmucosal) can be combined with low dose NSAID therapy such as meloxicam (0.025 mg/kg) for 2 or 3 days following traumatic injury or surgery.

Example Protocol

Premedication with medetomidine (8.0 mcg/kg) + atropine (0.044 mg/kg) + hydromorphone (0.2 mg/kg) given intramuscularly 20 minutes before induction. Anesthetic induction is achieved with either ketamine, thiopental, or propofol given "to effect" intravenously. After induction, but before surgery, epidural administration of morphine (0.2 mg/kg) q.s. to 1 ml/4.5 kg with bupivacaine (0.5%) will provide intraoperative analgesia/anesthesia and smooth recovery if the injury was to the *pelvic limb*. An epidural dose of 0.2 mg/kg morphine combined with 2-5 mcg/kg of medetomidine and q.s. to 1 ml / 4.5 kg with sterile saline provides analgesia to the *thoracic limb* without the potential for local anesthetic-induced respiratory depression.

✓ Management of traumatic degloving pain in cats can be approached in a similar fashion as described for dogs with the appropriate species modification of dosages and techniques.

NOTE Refer to Section 2, Figure 2-1, Tables 2-1, 2-2, 2-3, 2-4, 2-5, 2-6, 2-7, 2-8, and 2-9 for drug dosages and Section 3 for applicable techniques.

⊙ See CD for demonstration of Epidural Anesthesia (Video 3-1), Epidural Catheter Placement (Video 3-2), Brachial Plexus Nerve Block (Video 3-3), and other Regional Nerve Block (Video 3-4, 3-6, and 3-9), techniques.

Perianal Fistula

Anticipated Degree of Pain

Moderate

✓ A component of chronic pain is likely present in these patients.

Preemptive Analgesic Medications

✓ NSAIDs or opioids may be given before anesthesia or as part of the premedication protocol.

Regional Analgesic Technique

✓ Epidural placement of opioids or local anesthetics after induction of anesthesia will reduce the amount of afferent painful stimuli associated with surgery and can help prevent post operative straining.

Postoperative Analgesic Medications

✓ The epidural administration of a local anesthetic (especially bupivacaine) often provides good analgesia for 3 to 6 hours following surgery.

✓ Additional opioids or NSAIDs may be administered if the patient appears uncomfortable.

Dispensable Analgesic Medications

✓ Oral NSAIDs such as carprofen (4 mg/kg once a day) are usually adequate for dispensable analgesia. Oral opioid preparations such as morphine or butorphanol tablets may provide additional pain relief. Proprietary preparation such as acetaminophen with codeine #4 or Percocet tablets can be used in dogs as well.

Example Protocol

Premedication with acepromazine (0.05 mg/kg) + atropine (0.044 mg/kg) + morphine (0.5 mg/kg) given intramuscularly 20 minutes before induction with either ketamine, thiopental, or propofol given "to effect" intravenously. Anesthetic maintenance is accomplished with halothane or isoflurane. After induction, but before surgery, the epidural administration of morphine (0.2 mg/kg) q.s. to 1 ml / 4.5 kg with bupivacaine (0.5%) and 1 mg/kg of ketamine will provide intraoperative analgesia/anesthesia while reducing the potential for central hypersensitization.

NOTE Refer to Section 2, Figure 2-1, Tables 2-1, 2-2, 2-3, 2-4, 2-5, 2-6, 2-7, 2-8, and 2-9 for drug dosages and Section 3 for applicable techniques.

⊙ See CD for demonstration of Epidural Anesthesia (Video 3-1).

Ear Canal Ablation

Anticipated Degree of Pain

Moderate to Severe

Preemptive Analgesic Medications

✓ Injectable opioids (e.g., hydromorphone or morphine) and NSAIDs (e.g., carprofen) given 1-2 days in advance may help reduce the amount of postoperative analgesics required. NSAIDs should not be given with corticosteroid therapy. In some patients a fentanyl patch can be applied 24-36 hours prior to surgery.

Regional Analgesic Technique

✓ Local infiltration deep to the surgical incision using 2 mg/kg bupivacaine and 2 mg/kg lidocaine diluted with an equal volume of saline placed in a "U" pattern rostral, ventral and caudal to the external ear canal can be employed following induction of anesthesia and before initiation of surgery.

Postoperative Analgesic Medications

✓ Injectable opioid analgesics are usually efficacious for relieving pain associated with aural surgery. Addition of injectable or oral NSAIDs may enhance the analgesic effects of opioids and are efficacious against pain originating from inflammation and swelling.

✔ Within 3-5 hours post surgery a Lidoderm® patch in the shape of a "V" can be placed over the surgical incision site. Lidocaine patches can be left in place for only 12 h and then must be removed to prevent toxicity.

✔ Alternatively a sterile fenestrated catheter can be placed within the surgical incision in a "U" shape pattern and connected to an elastomeric reservoir (Pain Buster®) filled with lidocaine. This device can deliver a continuous infusion of local anesthetic for up to 5 days post surgery (Figure 4-1).

Dispensable Analgesic Medications

✔ Oral NSAIDs such as carprofen (4 mg/kg, once daily) or meloxicam (0.2 mg/kg initial dose followed by 0.1 mg/kg thereafter, once daily) are the most widely recommended dispensable analgesics for treatment of pain associated with aural surgery in dogs. Additional analgesia may be provided with morphine or butorphanol tablets given in combination with the oral NSAID. Concurrent glucocorticoid and NSAID therapy should not occur. A washout period of several days is recommended when switching from a short acting steroid to an NSAID and from one NSAID to another.

Example Protocol

Premedication with acepromazine (0.05 mg/kg) + hydromorphone (0.2 mg/kg) + atropine (0.044 mg/kg) given intramuscularly 20 minutes before induction with either ketamine, thiopental, or propofol given "to effect" intravenously. Anesthetic maintenance is accomplished with halothane or isoflurane. Postoperative analgesia is provided with morphine (0.5 mg/kg) or an NSAID. Buprenorphine or butorphanol may be added to the NSAID if necessary. Non-pharmacologic techniques such as cold packing the ear immediately following surgery may provide additional relief from discomfort associated with swelling and inflammation. This can be done as long as the patient will tolerate it.

✔ Management of aural surgical pain in cats can be approached in a similar fashion as described for dogs with the appropriate species modification of dosages and techniques.

NOTE Refer to Section 2, Figure 2-1, Tables 2-1, 2-2, 2-3, 2-4, 2-5, 2-6, 2-7, and 2-8 for drug dosages.

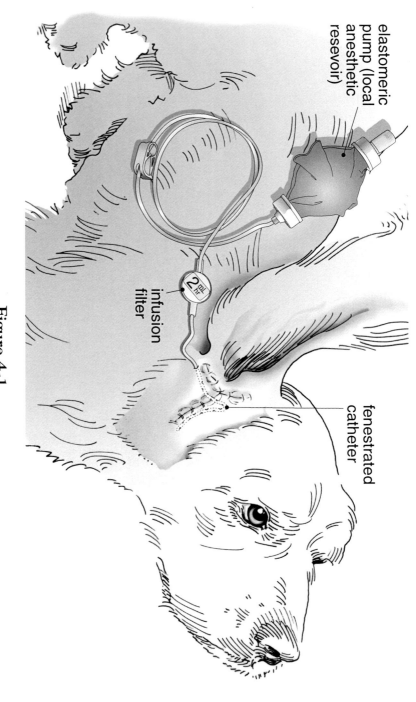

elastomeric
pump (local
anesthetic
resevoir)

infusion
filter

2 mL hr

fenestrated
catheter

Figure 4-1
Infiltration analgesia following total ear canal ablation (TECA) with continuous
infusion of local anesthetic by an elastomeric pump (Pain Buster®)

Common Feline Procedures

Declaw

Anticipated Degree of Pain

Moderate to Severe

✔ The level of pain experienced by any particular patient is a function of surgical technique and the animal's pain tolerance.

Preemptive Analgesic Medications

✔ Oral or injectable NSAIDs may be effective preemptive analgesics when given before surgery.

✔ Premedication with alpha$_2$ adrenergic agonists, opioids, and other analgesic drugs may reduce anesthetic and postoperative analgesic requirements.

Regional Analgesic Techniques

✔ Local infiltration may provide some degree of analgesia following surgery. A ring block around the limb proximal to the site of surgery can provide good analgesia.

✔ The use of laser surgical technique appears to result in less immediate post operative pain and discomfort.

✔ Distal block of the superficial branches of the radial nerve, the median nerve, and the dorsal and palmar branches of the ulnar nerve (3 point block) provide good analgesia for onychectomy surgery and may result in less bleeding than when a complete ring block technique is performed.

✔ Direct application of bupivacaine to the exposed digit (splash block) has been associated with increased pain behavior in some cats.

Postoperative Analgesic Medications

✔ Injectable carprofen (1-2 mg/kg SC once only) or ketoprofen (1-2 mg/kg, SC), opioids such as buprenorphine (0.01-0.02 mg/kg, SC, IV, or transmucosal) and/or adjunctive drugs such as alpha$_2$ adrenergic agonists all may be used to reduce the pain and stress following surgery.

Dispensable Analgesic Medications

✓ Low dose NSAID therapy (e.g., meloxicam, 0.1 mg/kg initial dose, PO) can be dispensed for treatment of postoperative pain (limited to 2 to 3 days in cats). Additional analgesia may be provided with butorphanol tablets (1.0 mg/kg, PO) or transmucosal buprenorphine administration (0.01-0.02 mg/kg) given every 8 hours. Buprenorphine can be accurately dosed at home by preloading drug into an insulin syringe for the pet owner to administer.

Example Protocol

Anesthesia is accomplished with medetomidine (35.0 mcg/kg) + butorphanol (0.2 mg/kg) + ketamine (5.0-10.0 mg/kg) given intramuscularly. Additional administration of halothane or isoflurane may be necessary. A distal radial/ulnar/median nerve block can provide intraoperative and postoperative pain control often eliminating the need for supplemental inhalation anesthetic administration. Additional postoperative analgesia can be provided by butorphanol (0.2 mg/kg, IM), hydromorphone (0.1 mg/kg, IM), buprenorphine (0.01-0.02 mg/kg, IM or transmucosal), or a fentanyl patch (25 mcg/hr patch).

NOTE Refer to Section 2, Figure 2-1, Tables 2-1, 2-2, 2-3, 2-4, 2-5, 2-6, 2-7, and 2-8 for drug dosages and Section 3 for applicable techniques.

⊙ See CD for demonstration of Radial/Ulnar/Median Nerve Block (Video 3-4) and Infiltrative Block (Video 3-7) techniques.

Ovariohysterectomy
Anticipated Degree of Pain
Mild to Severe

✓ The level of pain experienced by a particular patient is a function of surgical technique and the animal's pain tolerance.

Preemptive Analgesic Medications

✓ Premedication with alpha$_2$ adrenergic agonists, opioids, and other analgesic drugs often reduces anesthetic and postoperative analgesic requirements.

Regional Analgesic Techniques

✓ Regional nerve blocks are typically not performed for routine abdominal surgery.

✓ Intraperitoneal local anesthetics have been administered for laparoscopic and laparotomy procedures.

✓ Infiltration of the incision site with local anesthetic may provide postoperative analgesia. Lidocaine or bupivacaine can be combined with epinephrine (1:200,000) to help prolong block. A 1.5 mg/kg dose of bupivacaine (0.5% solution) diluted 1:1 with normal saline solution can provide enough volume. The block may last several hours.

Postoperative Analgesic Medications

✓ Injectable opioids and analgesic adjuvant drugs such as alpha$_2$ adrenergic agonists and other sedatives can be used to reduce pain and stress following OHE surgery.

Dispensable Analgesic Medications

✓ Oral meloxicam (0.1 mg/kg initial dose followed by 0.025 mg/kg q 24 hrs) can be combined with oral butorphanol or transmucosal buprenorphine for 2-3 days.

Example Protocol

Anesthesia is achieved with medetomidine (35.0 mcg/kg) + butorphanol (0.2 mg/kg) + ketamine (5.0-10.0 mg/kg) given together intramuscularly). Additional administration of low concentrations of halothane or isoflurane may be required. Postoperative analgesia is enhanced by butorphanol (0.2 mg/kg, IM), hydromorphone (0.1 mg/kg, IM) or buprenorphine (0.01-0.02 mg/kg, IM or transmucosal) administration.

NOTE Refer to Section 2, Figure 2-1, Tables 2-1, 2-2, 2-3, 2-4, 2-5, 2-7, and 2-8 for drug dosages.

Castration

Anticipated Degree of Pain

Mild to Moderate

✓ The level of pain experienced by any particular patient is a function of surgical technique and the animal's pain tolerance.

Preemptive Analgesic Medications

✓ Premedication with alpha$_2$ adrenergic agonists, opioids, and other analgesic drugs may reduce anesthetic and postoperative analgesic requirements.

Regional Analgesic Technique

✓ Regional nerve blocks are typically not performed for routine castration procedures.

Postoperative Analgesic Medications

✓ Injectable opioids and analgesic adjunctive drugs such as alpha$_2$ adrenergic agonists and other sedatives can be used to reduce pain and stress following castration.

Dispensable Analgesic Medications

✓ Additional analgesia may be provided at home for 2 to 3 days with butorphanol tablets or oral NSAIDs such as meloxicam.

Example Protocol

Premedication with medetomidine (35.0 mcg/kg body weight) + butorphanol (0.2 mg/kg) + ketamine (5.0-10.0 mg/kg) given together intramuscularly. A low concentration of halothane or isoflurane may be required to supplement anesthetic action. Postoperative analgesia can be provided with butorphanol (0.2 mg/kg, SC) hydromorphone (0.1 mg/kg, SC) or buprenorphine (0.01-0.02 mg/kg IM or transmucosal), when required. NSAID therapy with either ketoprofen (1-2 mg/kg, SC) carprofen (1-2 mg/kg, SC) or meloxicam (0.1 mg/kg, SC or PO) may also be effective for mild to moderate discomfort during the first day following surgery.

NOTE Refer to Section 2, Figure 2-1, Tables 2-1, 2-3, 2-4, 2-5, 2-7, and 2-8 for drug dosages.

Section 5

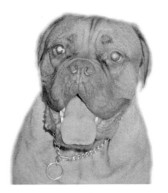

Managing Chronic Pain in Dogs and Cats

Chronic Pain

✔ Chronic pain is pain that persists beyond the usual course of an acute disease or beyond a reasonable time required for an injury to heal.

♥ Pain can persist even though all signs of tissue injury have disappeared.

✔ Chronic pain is characterized by abnormal activity within the peripheral and/or central nervous system.

✔ Sensitization of peripheral nociceptors or central nervous system sensitization "wind up" causes abnormal processing of afferent stimuli. Continued afferent activity may lead to nervous system memory resulting in pain originating from nervous tissue, apart from the original injury (neuropathic pain). (See Tables 5-1 and 5-2).

✔ Chronic pain is seldom permanently alleviated by analgesics alone, but may respond to drugs classified as analgesic adjuvants such as the tricyclic antidepressants, tranquilizers, GABA receptor agonists, and NMDA receptor antagonists. (See Table 2-5 in Section 2 for specific drugs and recommended dosages.)

Table 5-1
Possible Mechanisms for Developing Chronic Pain

Sensitization of nociceptors
Spread of excitation from damaged neurons to adjacent undamaged neurons (both nociceptors and low threshold receptors) that normally subserve mild sensations such as non-noxious warmth or pressure (allodynia).
Expansion of the peripheral receptive fields of dorsal horn neurons
Increased excitability in populations of neurons within central nociceptive pathways
Diminished activity of endogenous inhibitory mechanisms leading to the reduced inhibition of excitability within nociceptive pathways

✔ The exact mechanisms for development of chronic pain in a given patient are often poorly understood.

✔ Many of the drugs that appear efficacious for treating chronic pain have actions at specific receptor systems involved in nervous system transmission and action potential conduction. A common theme which adequately describes the mechanism of all analgesic drugs is yet to be described.

Table 5-2 Examples of Common Conditions Which May Lead to Chronic Pain	
CONDITION	EXAMPLE
Malignancy	Osteosarcoma
Chronic inflammatory disorders	Chronic otitis
Chronic orthopedic disorders	Cervical intervertebral disk disease
Chronic soft tissue injury	Degloving injuries
Nervous tissue injury	Phantom limb pain

✔ Not all patients with the above conditions will develop symptoms of altered nervous system processing.

✔ It is difficult to treat chronic pain effectively. Therefore, an aggressive treatment strategy when symptoms first appear may have the best outcome.

Treatment of Chronic Pain

✓ When altered CNS processing of afferent information becomes problematic, endogenous hypoalgesic mechanisms often become less effective. Consequently alternative analgesic therapy becomes increasingly important for providing relief. Drug therapies include tricyclic antidepressants (e.g., clomipramine), anticonvulsants (e.g., gabapentin), NMDA receptor antagonists (e.g., ketamine), and other drugs which are not typically classified as analgesics (Figure 5-1). Experimentation with several different medications or combinations may be necessary to find an effective therapy.

✓ Alternatives to drug therapy such as acupuncture, physical therapy, and neuroablative techniques have not been widely utilized in veterinary medicine to date.

✓ Assessment of analgesic efficacy is usually subjective and varies among observers. Pain intensity assessment scales and pain relief scales currently used on veterinary patients for acute pain are of limited use for chronic pain conditions. Owners may be best equipped to monitor changes in the animal's level of activity, mood, and appetite, all of which may be indirect measures of pain relief. However, owners may become biased when expectations of pain relief are established.

♥ The clinical usefulness of any pain management protocol may be limited by the adverse effects associated with its chronic use. Careful dose titration, substitution of other drugs within the same class, and substitution of drugs from other classes may reduce the incidence of side effects. The occurrence of side effects may vary between individuals and a bad experience with a protocol in one patient should not completely discourage its trial in another. The owner should be counseled on the difficulty of managing chronic pain and be informed that several different approaches may be tried.

✓ The Oxford Pain Chart can be the client's daily monitor of the efficacy of the pain management plan. (Figure 5-2).

✓ Systematic reviews of analgesic drugs and techniques for treating chronic pain clinically in dogs and cats are not available. Much of the evidence of hypoalgesic efficacy is based upon anecdotal reports.

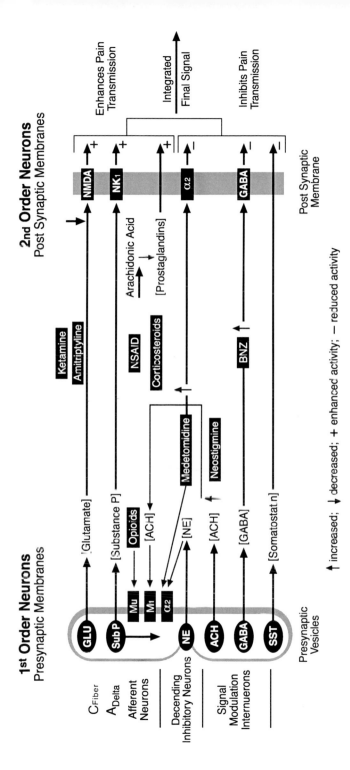

Figure 5-1

Neurotransmitters, receptors, and mechanisms of analgesic drug action in the dorsal horn of the spinal cord

112

Name _____

Treatment Week _____

Please fill in this chart each evening before going to bed. Record your estimation of your pet's pain intensity and the amount of pain relief. If your pet had any side-effects please note them in the side-effects box.

Date							
Pain Intensity How bad was your pet's pain today?	Severe						
	Moderate						
	Mild						
	None						
Pain relief How much pain relief has the medication given your pet today?	Complete						
	Good						
	Moderate						
	Slight						
	None						
Side-effects Has the treatment upset your pet in any way?							

How effective was the treatment this week?

Poor   Fair   Good   Very Good   Excellent

please circle one choice

Figure 5-2

An adaptation of the Oxford Pain Chart for assessment of chronic pain in pets

113

Guidelines for Chronic Pain Management

✓ Animals presenting for pain or discomfort associated with a previous injury should be thoroughly evaluated for reoccurrence of the same injury (or development of a new one) before analgesic treatment is begun.

✓ Pain management strategies for chronic pain are not a substitute for a complete diagnostic evaluation and correct medical diagnosis. Pain may be a symptom of a serious underlying condition and, if left untreated, may cause permanent injury or death to the patient.

✓ Initially conventional analgesics or techniques should be used in both chronic and acute pain. If for example analgesics or rehabilitation therapy relieve pain adequately with tolerable or controllable side effects, there is little reason to initiate treatment with analgesic adjuvant drugs or techniques.

✓ A guideline for the treatment of chronic cancer pain is provided by the World Health Organization (WHO) (Figure 5-3).

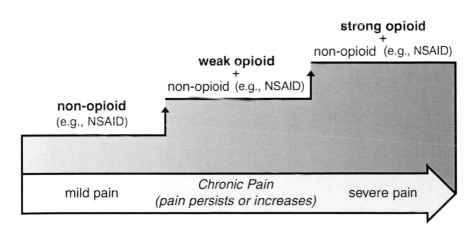

Figure 5-3
Schematic of World Health Organization ladder
for cancer pain management

✓ If long-term treatment with analgesic drugs is deemed appropriate, it may be prudent to collect baseline biochemical data and blood cell counts, followed by periodic rechecks to monitor for side effects associated with long-term analgesic therapy.

✓ Many drug protocols for the treatment of chronic pain are extra-label or off-label uses. A degree of liability is incurred by the veterinarian when these drugs are used in a manner for which they were not intended. The owner should be informed of this when consent for treatment is obtained.

✓ The therapeutic goal for pain management of terminally ill patients, or patients with intractable pain secondary to an undiagnosable condition, should be to improve the quality of life for the patient while minimizing adverse reactions.

Common Chronic Pain Syndromes

Osteoarthritic Pain

✓ Osteoarthritis is the most common cause of chronic pain in companion animals.

✓ A typical patient suffering from chronic pain is an older animal with a history of reluctance to rise, jump, or run (especially after periods of inactivity). The pain may start as an occasional soreness or stiffness following vigorous activity. It usually progresses to daily discomfort and quality of life is affected.

✓ Administration of analgesic drugs is only a part of a complete treatment plan for osteoarthritis. Weight reduction, controlled exercise, disease modifying agents (eg.: glucosamine or chondroitin sulfate) acupuncture, and surgery may each have a role in the treatment of this chronic condition.

Pain Management Strategies

✓ Treatment usually begins with recommendations for weight loss, implementation of an appropriate exercise regime, use of glucosamine and chondroitin sulfate products and the occasional administration of NSAIDs for control of pain associated with intermittent flair ups.

❤ When initiating therapy with NSAIDs, always try to "titrate down" to the animal's minimal effective dose.

✓ Daily administration of oral NSAIDs (e.g., carprofen, 4 mg/kg once daily or 2 mg/kg BID) is often necessary in more advanced stages of arthritis to make the discomfort tolerable and restore a level of normal behavior.

✓ In some cases, addition of oral opioids, other analgesic adjuvant drugs, or surgery may be required.

✓ When switching from an NSAID because of concern for developing toxicity in the patient, a "washout" period of several days is recommended before reinstating NSAID therapy with a second drug.

✓ If a switch to another NSAID is being made without concerns of toxicity, but rather based on a search for improved efficacy, the period between discontinuing the first NSAID and initiating the second NSAID may be quite variable depending on the specific NSAIDs involved and the underlying general health of organ systems at risk for NSAID induced toxicity (i.e., gastrointestinal tract, kidneys, cardiovascular system).

✓ If a "washout" period is not possible, the co-administration of a protectant such as misoprostil (2-5 mcg/kg, PO BID) for the first few days of administration of the new NSAID may be helpful. However, development of adverse effects when two NSAIDs interact may be multifactorial and difficult to predict and prevent.

✓ During "washout" periods pain can often be effectively controlled by careful regulation of exercise, acupuncture therapy 2 to 3 times a week and/or oral morphine (0.5 mg/kg, BID) therapy. Alternatively, a combination of an oral opioid and acetaminophen (e.g., Percocet®) tablets) can be given two to three times a day.

NOTE See Section 2, Tables 2-4, 2-5, 2-7, 2-8, 2-9 for specific drugs and dosages.

Osteosarcoma-related Pain

✓ Pain associated with neoplasia is often under treated in veterinary medicine. Tumor growth is usually gradual and subtle changes in pain intensity are difficult to detect.

✓ Expect that some degree of pain will accompany interference with normal use of the body part affected by the neoplasm.

✓ Standard pain management protocols for the treatment of cancer pain follow the World Health Organization's ladder (see Figure 5-3).

♥ Treatment of terminal patients should be governed by the ability of the veterinarian to provide a good quality of life. Quality of life must be of paramount concern to the owner and the veterinarian.

Pain Management Strategies

✓ Amputation, radiation therapy, bisphosphonates, or other palliative treatments may significantly reduce the pain associated with the progression of osteosarcoma.

✓ Analgesic protocols for the treatment of pain associated with cancer begin with oral administration of NSAIDs. In the very early stages of the disease, treatment may only be needed during episodes of pain. As the disease progresses, daily NSAID treatment may be necessary.

✓ When the pain becomes uncontrollable with NSAIDs, weak oral opioids may help make the pain tolerable. These combinations are usually well tolerated, but sedation, constipation, and other side effects may dictate the dose. Tolerance may develop to some side effects while others worsen during the course of therapy.

✓ When the pain becomes intense and likely has a neuropathic component, oral morphine or tramadol, or transdermal opioids may be combined with a NSAID. This phase of treatment is associated with end stages of the disease and side effects may increase. Adding adjuvant analgesic drugs such as amantidine, gabapentin or amitriptyline to treat abnormal neuroprocessing (hyperalgesia or allodynia) or utilizing techniques such as acupuncture, may be beneficial at this stage of therapy.

NOTE See Section 2, Tables 2-1, 2-4, 2-5, 2-6, 2-7, 2-8, and 2-9 for specific drugs and dosages.

Central Neuropathic Pain

✔ Chronic neck and back pain may be caused by intervertebral disk disease, nerve root entrapment, neoplasia, and infection or inflammation.

♥ Analgesic administration should not be considered a replacement for appropriate surgical treatment of neck or back lesions.

✔ A significant number of animals with lesions in and around nervous tissues suffer with neuropathic pain. These animals may display an increased intensity of pain to mild noxious stimuli (hyperalgesia) and respond in an exaggerated manner to stimuli which are not normally painful (allodynia).

✔ Analgesic drugs should not be withheld based upon a fear of worsening of the injury due to increased activity. Analgesics typically reduce the degree of pain but do not alleviate it completely. The patient should not be required to suffer. Instead the owner should be instructed to strictly confine the animal and only allow controlled activity. The severe consequences of failing to adhere to these recommendations should be emphasized to the owner.

♠ NSAIDs, particularly aspirin, should not be administered if spinal surgery is planned in the immediate future because of the increased risk of intraoperative hemorrhage.

Pain Management Strategies

♥ The concurrent use of NSAIDs and corticosteroids is not encouraged because of the increased chance of gastrointestinal ulceration. Use of H_2 antagonists, $H^+K^+ATPase$ inhibitors, sucralfate, and prostaglandin analogs such as misoprostol may help reduce the occurrence of ulceration associated with long term prostaglandin synthesis inhibition by NSAIDs.

✔ Oral or transdermal opioids are useful in the treatment of pain accompanying intervertebral disk disease. If the response to opioids is unsatisfactory, adjuvant drugs such as amantidine, gabapentin, amitriptyline and low dose ketamine may help reduce central hypersensitization and neuropathic pain.

NOTE See Section 2, Tables 2-1, 2-4, 2-5, 2-6, 2-7, 2-8, and 2-9 for specific drugs and dosages.

Chronic Otitis Pain

✔ Pain from chronic otitis media is a common condition. Historically, analgesic administration has not always been a part of the treatment plan.

✔ Scratching, pawing, or guarding the head or ears should be considered signs of pain and discomfort.

✔ Chronic exposure of nociceptors to inflammatory mediators may increase the sensitivity of the nociceptors (peripheral sensitization), and cause intense and exaggerated responses to stimuli which are usually innocuous (e.g., cleaning with a cotton-tipped applicator).

✔ Animals that have undergone surgical removal of auricular tissue in an attempt to treat otitis often display intense distress following surgery. There are both acute and chronic components to their pain.

✔ NSAIDs may be useful in conditions associated with chronic inflammation since the analgesic effects are mediated in part by their inhibition of synthesis of inflammatory mediators.

Pain Management Strategies

✔ Oral NSAIDs may provide relief from pain associated with the irritation and inflammation of otitis. Opioid therapy may be useful following vigorous cleaning of the ear canal.

✔ Anesthetic management of these patients for surgical removal of the ear canal can be improved by the addition of analgesic pre-medications and intraoperative analgesic drugs such as opioids, alpha$_2$ adrenergic agonists, and ketamine.

✔ Pain associated behaviors (guarding, scratching, pawing) may continue despite the apparent improvement in the condition of the ear. Although the mechanisms of abnormal cranial nerve pain processing are less understood than spinal cord pain processing, the possibility of central wind-up or a neuropathic component of chronic pain with this condition should not be dismissed.

NOTE See Section 2, Figure 2-1, Tables 2-1, 2-3, 2-4, 2-5, 2-6, 2-7, 2-8, and 2-9 for specific drugs and dosages.

Section **6**

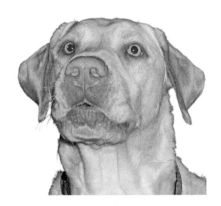

Implementing a Pain Management Program in Clinical Practice

Components of a Successful Pain Management Program

1. Ensure a strong practice commitment to minimizing pain.

2. Adopt a team approach involving veterinarians, technicians, and staff.

3. Provide pain management education for all practice personnel and owners.

4. Encourage continuous program assessment and improvement.

Recommendations for Assessment and Management of Pain in Clinical Practice

1. Assess all patients for the presence and intensity of pain or distress.

2. Record results in a manner that facilitates regular reassessment and follow-up.

3. Determine and assure staff competency in pain assessment and management.

4. Address pain assessment and management during the orientation of all new staff.

5. Write protocols for different case types encountered in daily practice. These should be an extension of the hospital's standard of care for patients. Evidence-based protocols should be adopted when available. Remember that individual responses to therapies can vary widely, requiring protocols to be individualized.

6. Establish policies and procedures which support appropriate dispensing of effective pain medications.

7. Ensure that pain does not interfere with patient recovery and rehabilitation.

8. Educate owners about pain assessment and management.

9. Document effectiveness of pain interventions in both hospitalized and discharged patients (see Oxford Pain Chart).

10. Plan for patient needs in relation to anticipated side effects associated with pain management plan.

11. Use consent forms and client education literature to emphasize the practice's commitment to pain management.

12. Revise pain management protocols periodically to reflect advances in veterinary pain management.

✓ The practice should adopt a standardized assessment tool (such as the visual analog scale or numerical rating scale) that can be used by all team members on a routine basis. It should be remembered that all scales have shortcomings related to variability, accuracy, and ease of use. However, the most important aspect in using any pain assessment scheme is its value in focusing the caregiver's and owner's attention on patient pain and distress.

✓ When beginning a pain management program, practitioners may find perioperative pain easier to manage effectively. Chronic pain associated with longstanding or CNS disease often presents challenges to even the most experienced clinician and may require unusual approaches not commonly utilized in most practices.

✓ Specialists with an interest in pain management include anesthesiologists, surgeons, oncologists, internists, and clinical pharmacologists. Consultation may be warranted when unusual clinical cases are treated.

✓ Several academic referral centers within North America have pain management consultation services available.

✓ The recently established International Veterinary Academy of Pain Management can be contacted for more information and additional materials concerning the implementation of pain management protocols and hospital programs.

Appendix

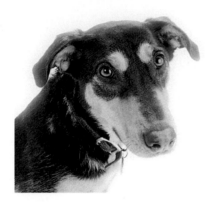

Drugs and Sources

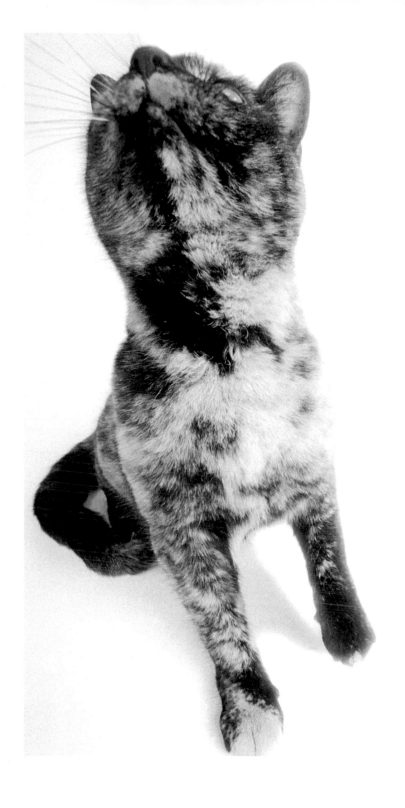

Drugs and Sources

Acetaminophen

Trade Name Tylenol, and numerous generic products available
Tablet Size 325 mg, 500 mg, 650 mg
Also available as chewable tablets, caplets, gel capsules, and elixir

Amantadine

Trade Name Symmetrel
Concentration 10 mg/mL
Capsule size 100 mg
Available in numerous generic products

Amitriptyline

Trade Name Elavil
Tablet Size 10 mg, 25 mg, 50 mg, 75 mg, 100 mg, 150 mg
Available in numerous generic products

Aspirin

Numerous generic products available
Tablet Size 65 mg, 81 mg, 325 mg, 500 mg
Also available in formulations buffered with aluminum and/or
magnesium salts

Bupivacaine Hydrochloride

Trade Name Marcaine Hydrochloride
Concentration 5 mg/mL
Supplied as 10 mL, 30 mL, 50 mL/vial
Company Sanofi Winthrop Pharmaceuticals, New York, NY 10016

Buprenorphine Hydrochloride (Schedule V)

Trade Name Buprenex Injectable
Concentration 0.3 mg/mL
Supplied as 1 mL/ampule (5 ampules/box)
Manufacturer Reckitt and Coleman Products Ltd.
Hull, England HU87DS
Distributor Reckitt and Coleman Pharmaceuticals Ltd.
Richmond, VA 23235
Web site http://www.reccolpharm.com

Butorphanol Tartrate (Schedule IV)

Trade Name Torbugesic-SA
Concentration 2 mg/mL
Supplied as 10 mL/vial
Company Fort Dodge Laboratories, Inc., Fort Dodge, IA 50501
Web site http://www.ahp.com/fort_dodge/fort_dodge.asp

Trade Name Torbugesic
Concentration 10 mg/mL
Supplied as 50 mL/vial
Company Fort Dodge Laboratories, Inc., Fort Dodge, IA 50501
Web site http://www.ahp.com/fort_dodge/fort_dodge.asp

Trade Name Torbutrol
Tablet Size 1 mg, 5 mg, 10 mg
Supplied as 100/bottle
Company Fort Dodge Laboratories, Inc., Fort Dodge, IA 50501
Web site http://www.ahp.com/fort_dodge/fort_dodge.asp

Carprofen

Trade Name Rimadyl
Caplet and Tablet Size 25 mg, 75 mg, 100 mg
Supplied as 30, 100, 250/bottle
Injectable formulation Concentration 50 mg/ml
Supplied as 10 ml multidose vial
Company Pfizer Animal Health, New York City, NY 10017
Web site http://www.Pfizer.com/ah

Codeine (Schedule III)

Trade Name Codeine Phosphate available in numerous generic
products
Tablet Size 15 mg, 30 mg, 60 mg

Deracoxib

Trade Name Deramaxx
Tablet Size 25 mg, 100 mg
Supplied as 7, 30, or 90/bottle
Company Novartis Animal Health, Greensboro, NC 27408
Web site http://www.deramaxx.com

Etodolac

Trade Name Etogesic
Tablet Size 150 mg, 300 mg
Supplied as 100, 250/bottle
Company Fort Dodge Laboratories, Fort Dodge, IA 50501
Web site http://www.ahp.com/fort_dodge/.asp

Fentanyl Citrate (Schedule II)

Label Name Fentanyl Citrate Injection, USP
Concentration 50 mcg/mL
Supplied as 50 mL/vial
Company Wyeth-Ayerst / Elkins-Sinn, Philadelphia, PA 19101
Web site www.wyeth.com

Fentanyl Transdermal System (Schedule II)

Trade Name Duragesic
Patch Size 25 µg/hr, 50 µg/hr, 75 µg/hr, 100 µg/hr
Manufacturer ALZA Corporation, Palo Alto, CA 94304
Web site http://mimi.zoomedia.com/alza/
Distributor Janssen Pharmaceutica, Inc., Titusville, NJ 08560
Web site http://us.janssen.com

Gabapentin

Trade Name Neurontin
Tablet Size 100 mg, 300 mg, 400 mg
Supplied as 100/bottle
Company Pfizer Animal Health, New York City, NY 10017
Web site http://www.Pfizer.com/ah

Hydromorphone Hydrochloride (Schedule II)

Trade Name Dilaudid
Concentration 2 mg/ mL
Supplied as 20 mL/vial
Company Knoll Pharmaceutical Company, Mount Olive, NJ 07828
Web site http://www.basf.com/knoll/index2.html

Trade Name Hydromorphone
Concentration 2 mg/mL
Supplied as 20 mL/vial
Company Wyeth-Ayerst / Elkins-Sinn, Philadelphia, PA 19101
Web site www.wyeth.com

Ketoprofen

Trade Name Ketofen
Concentration 100 mg/mL
Supplied as 50 mL, 100 mL/vial
Company Fort Dodge Laboratories, Fort Dodge, IA 50501
Web site http://www.ahp.com/fort_dodge/fort_dodge.asp

Trade Name Orudis
Capsule Size 25 mg, 50 mg, 75 mg
Supplied as 100, 500/bottle
Company Wyeth-Ayerst, Philadelphia, PA 19101
Web site www.wyeth.com

Trade Name Anafen (Canada)
Concentration 10 mg/mL, 100 mg/mL
Supplied as 20 mL, 50 mL, 100 mL/vial
Company Rhone Merieux Canada, Inc.,Victoriaville, Quebec G6P 1B1

Trade Name Anafen (Canada)
Tablet Size 5 mg, 10 mg, 20 mg
Supplied as foil blister packets with 10 tablets/strip (one strip/packet)
Company Rhone Merieux Canada, Inc.,Victoriaville, Quebec G6P 1B1

Lidocaine

Trade Name Xylocaine
Concentration 20 mg/mL
Supplied as 20 mL/vial
Company Astra Labs, Inc.,Westborough, MA 01581
Web site http://www.astrazeneca.com

Trade Name Lidocaine HCL 2%
Concentration 20 mg/mL
Supplied as 100 mL/vial
Company Western Veterinary Supply, Inc., Portersville, CA 93257

Lidocaine Cream

Trade Name ELA Max Cream
Concentration 4% liposomal lidocaine
Supplied as 5 and 30 g tubes
Company Ferndale Laboratories, Ferndale, Michigan 48220
Web site http://www.ferndalelabs.com

Lidocaine Patch

Trade Name Lidoderm
Concentration 5% (700 mg)
Patch Size (10 x 14 cm patch)
Company Endo Laboratories, Chadds Ford, PA 19317
Web Site http://www.endo.com

EMLA (Lidocaine-Prilocaine)

Trade Name EMLA Cream
Concentration lidocaine 25 mg/mL and prilocaine 25 mg/mL
Supplied as 5 g tube (1 or 5 tubes/box) or 30 g tube (1 tube/box)
Manufacturer Astra Pharm, Sodertalje, Sweden
Web site http://www.astrazeneca.com
Distributor Astra USA, Inc., Westborough, MA 01581
Web site http://www.astrazeneca.com

Medetomidine Hydrochloride

Trade Name Domitor
Concentration 1 mg/mL
Supplied as 10 mL/vial
Manufacturer Orion Corporation, Espoo, Finland
Distributor Pfizer Animal Health, New York City, NY 10017
Web site http://www.Pfizer.com/ah

Meloxicam

Trade Name Metacam
Concentration 1.5 mg/mL oral suspension
Supplied as 10, 32, 100 mL/bottle
Manufacturer Boehringer Ingelheim

Distributor Merial Ltd. Duluth, GA 30096-4640
Web site http://www.merial.com/main.html

Trade Name Metacam
Concentration 5 mg/mL injectable formulation
Supplied as 10 mL-vial
Manufacturer Boehringer Ingelheim
Distributor Merial Ltd. Duluth, GA 30096-4640
Web site http://www.merial.com/main.html

Mepivacaine Hydrochloride

Trade Name Carbocaine -V
Concentration 20 mg/mL
Supplied as 50 mL/vial
Manufacturer Abbott Laboratories, North Chicago, IL 60064
Web site http://www.abbott.com
Distributor Pfizer Animal Health, Kalamazoo, MI 49001
Web site http://www.Pfizer.com/ah

Morphine (Schedule II)

Trade Name Morphine Sulfate
Concentration 15 mg/mL
Supplied as 20 mL/vial
Company Wyeth-Ayerst / Elkins-Sinn, Philadelphia, PA 19101
Web site www.wyeth.com

Trade Name Astramorph PF (Preservative Free)
Concentration 1 mg/mL
Supplied as 10 mL/ampule (5 ampules/box)
Company Astra Labs, Inc., Westborough, MA 01581
Web site http://www.astrazeneca.com

Trade Name Morphine Sulfate
Tablet Size 15 mg, 30 mg
Numerous generic preparations available

Nerve locator

Trade Name Tracer III
Stimulus Range 0.5-5.0 Amps
Manufacturer Life-Tech Inc. Stafford, TX 77477-3995
Web site http://www.life-tech.com

Pain Buster

Pump Size 65-335 ml volume (0.5, 2, 4, 5 ml/h)
Manufacturer IFlow Corporation, Lake Forest, CA
Distributor DJ Orthopedics Inc.
Web Site http://www.donjoy.com

Pamidronate Disodium

Trade Name Aredia
Supplied as 30 mg vial
Manufacture Benvenue Laboratory
Distributor Bedford Laboratories, Bedford, OH 44146
Web site http://www.bedfordlabs.com/

Piroxicam

Trade Name Feldane
Capsule Size 10 and 20 mg
Available as numerous generic products

Tepoxalin

Trade Name Zubrin
Size 50, 100, 200 mg
Supplied as 100 doses/box
Company Schering-Plough Animal Health, Union, NJ 07083
Web site http://usa.spah.com/home.cfm

Tolfenamic Acid

Trade Name Tolfedine
Concentration 40 mg/ml
Supplied as 30 ml vial
Tablet Size 6 mg, 20 mg, 60 mg
Company Vetoquinol, Lavaltrie, Quebec J0K 1 H0

Tramadol

Trade Name Ultram, Tramal
Supplied as 50 mg tablets
Available in numerous generic products

Xylazine

Trade Name Rompun SA
Concentration 20 mg/mL
Supplied as 20 mL/vial
Company Miles Inc., Shawnee Mission, KS 66201

Numerous large animal Xylazine generic products are available

INDEX

Page numbers followed by an *f* indicate a figure;
page numbers followed by a *t* indicate a table

135

G

G protein, membrane-associated, 19

GABA receptor agonists, 109
    for chronic pain, 111

Gabapentin
    for central neuropathic pain,
      118
    dosages and indications for, 26t
    with hind limb amputation/
      fracture, 97
    for osteosarcoma-related pain, 117

Glucocorticoids
    dosages and indications for, 26t
    with ear canal ablation, 102

Glucosamine
    for osteoarthritic pain, 116
    for osteoarthritis, 115

H

Halothane
    with castration, 107
    with cruciate ligament repair, 95
    with declawing, 105
    with ear canal ablation, 102
    with exploratory laparotomy/
      cystotomy, 87
    with intervertebral disc
      disease, 94
    with ovariohysterectomy, 84

Hanging drop technique, 35

Head trauma
    degree of pain in, 78
    dispensable analgesic
      medications for, 78-79
    postoperative analgesics for, 78
    preemptive analgesic
      medications for, 78
    protocol for, 79
    regional analgesic techniques
      for, 78

Hind limb
    amputation of in dogs, 96-98
    weakness of with epidural
      injection, 42

Histamine-2 receptor (H_2)
    antagonists, 119
    for NSAID GI pathology, 22

H^+K^+ATPase inhibitors, 118

Hormonal opiate theory, 72

Huber point gauge, 37

Human contact, 12

Hydromorphone
    with castration, 85, 107
    with declawing, 104
    with degloving injury, 99
    with ear canal ablation, 101, 102
    for head trauma, 79
    with hind limb amputation/
      fracture, 96
    with ovariohysterectomy, 105
    recommended dosages and
      indications for, 16t
    routes for in dogs and cats, 28
    with thoracotomy, 92
    for traumatic injury, 77

Hydrotherapy, 71

Hyperalgesia, 2

Hyperesthesia, 2

Hyperthermia, 71

Hypoalgesia, 2

Hypothermia, 71

I

Idiopathic pain, 3

Imipramine, 93

Infiltrative block
    areas to be desensitized in, 56
    complications and
      contraindications in, 57
    with declawing, 104
    drugs and dosages in, 55
    materials needed in, 55
    technical skills in, 57
    technique in, 54-55

Infra-orbital nerve block, 50-51
    for dental cleaning with
      extractions, 81

Injections, 71

Intercostal nerve block
    anatomical landmarks for, 62
    complications and
      contraindications in, 61
    drugs and dosages in, 61
    materials needed in, 61
    technical skills for, 63
    technique in, 61
    with thoracotomy, 91

International Veterinary Academy
    of Pain Management, 122

analgesia/anesthesia, 58
ionotophoretic application of, 72
with ovariohysterectomy, 106
in radial/ulnar/median nerve
block, 47

Lidocaine patch, 30
with ear canal ablation, 102

Lidoderm patch, 102

Lipoxin, 22

Local anesthetics,
ionotophoretic application of, 72

Lumbosacral epidural space, 38-40

M

Magnetic field induction, 73

Magnets, 71

Mandibular nerve block, 52-53
for dental cleaning with
extractions, 81
for head trauma, 78

Massage therapy, 71

Maxillary nerve block
for dental cleaning with
extractions, 81
for head trauma, 78

Medetomidine
with castration, 107
with cruciate ligament repair, 95
with declawing, 104
with degloving injury, 99
for dental cleaning with
extractions, 82
dosages and indications to, 20t
with forelimb amputation/
fracture, 90
with hind limb amputation/
fracture, 97
in initial pain management, 77
with intervertebral disc
disease, 94
with ovariohysterectomy, 105
routes for in dogs and cats,
27, 28

Median nerve block, 45-47
with declawing, 104

Meloxicam
with castration, 107
with declawing, 104
for dental cleaning with
extractions, 81

dosages and indications for, 23t
with ear canal ablation, 102
with forelimb amputation/
fracture, 90
oral preparations of for dogs
and cats, 32t
with ovariohysterectomy, 106

Mepivacaine, 18t

Metacam oral suspension, 32t

Methadone, 16t

Mexilitine, 26t

Midazolam, 27, 28

Misoprostil
for NSAID GI pathology, 22
for osteoarthritic pain, 116

Modulation, 6

Morphine
with cruciate ligament repair, 95
with degloving injury, 99
with ear canal ablation, 101, 102
in epidural anesthesia, 37
in epidural catheterization, 41
with forelimb amputation/
fracture, 89, 90
with hind limb amputation/
fracture, 96, 97-98
with intervertebral disc
disease, 94
in intra-articular analgesia, 48
for intravenous constant rate
infusion, 67
oral preparations of, 33t
for osteoarthritic pain, 116
for osteosarcoma-related pain, 117
with perianal fistula, 100, 101
recommended dosages and
indications for, 16t
routes for in dogs and cats, 28
for traumatic injury, 77

Moxibustion, 71

Mu opioid agonists, 94

Muscle relaxants, 25

N

Needle insertion, 35

Neuroablative techniques, 111

Neuroendocrine stress response, 10-11

Neuroleptics, 25

Neurolytic techniques, 73

Neuropathic pain
  central, 119
  definition of, 3

Neurotransmitters, 112*f*

Nitric oxide, 22

NMDA receptor antagonists, 109
  as analgesic adjuvant agents, 25
  for chronic pain, 111
  with degloving injury, 98
  dosages and indications for, 26*t*

Nociception, 6

Nociceptive pain, 2

Nociceptor sensitization, surgery-
  induced peripheral, 10

Nonsteroidal antiinflammatory
  drugs (NSAIDs)
  with castration, 84-85, 107
  for central neuropathic pain, 118
  for chronic otitis pain, 119
  with cruciate ligament repair,
    94-95
  with declawing, 104
  with degloving injury, 99
  for dental cleaning with
    extractions, 81-82
  drug interactions of, 22
  with ear canal ablation, 101-102
  with exploratory laparotomy/
    cystotomy, 87
  with forelimb amputation/
    fracture, 88, 89-90
  for head trauma, 78-79
  with hind limb amputation/
    fracture, 97
  in initial pain management, 76
  with intervertebral disc
    disease, 93
  mechanisms of action of, 21
  oral preparations of, 32-33
  for osteoarthritic pain, 116
  for osteosarcoma-related pain, 117
  with ovariohysterectomy, 83
  with perianal fistula, 100
  preemptive, 10
  preemptive combinations of,
    27-28
  recommended dosages and
    indications for, 23-24*t*
  side effects, toxicity, and
    contraindications to, 21-22

with thoracotomy, 91

NSAIDs. *See* Nonsteroidal
  antiinflammatory drugs
  (NSAIDs)

Numby Stuff, 72

Numerical rating scale (NRS), 9, 122

O

Omeprazole, 22

OP1 receptor, 15

OP2 receptor, 15

OP3 receptor, 15

Opioid/acetaminophen
  preparations, oral, 33*t*

Opioid agonists
  dosages and indications for, 26*t*
  for head trauma, 78-79

Opioids. *See also specific agents*
  for acute pancreatitis, 79
  with castration, 84-85, 107
  for central neuropathic pain, 118
  for chronic otitis pain, 119
  with cruciate ligament repair,
    94-95
  with declawing, 104-105
  with degloving injury, 99
  for dental cleaning with
    extractions, 81
  drug interactions of, 15
  with ear canal ablation, 101
  endogenous, 12
  with exploratory laparotomy/
    cystotomy, 87
  with forelimb amputation/
    fracture, 89
  for head trauma, 78
  with hind limb amputation/
    fracture, 96-97
  in initial pain management, 76
  with intervertebral disc
    disease, 93
  mechanism of action of, 15
  oral, 33*t*
  for osteoarthritic pain, 116
  for osteosarcoma-related
    pain, 117
  with ovariohysterectomy,
    105-106
  with perianal fistula, 100
  preemptive, 10

with ovariohysterectomy,
83, 105-106
with perianal fistula, 100
with thoracotomy, 91

Rehabilitation therapy, 71
with cruciate ligament repair, 95

Respiratory rate, 8

Rimadyl, 32t

S

Sedative, 77

Segmented reflex activity, 4

Sensitization, 109

Sensory nerve, 7

Sensory nervous system, 4-7

Sodium bicarbonate, 19

Soft tissue injury, 77

Somatic pain, 3

Spinal cord
damage to with epidural
injection, 41
dorsal horn of, analgesic drug
action in, 112f
in pain modulation, 7

Spinal needle, 37

Spinocervical tract, 4

Spinomesencephalic tract, 4

Sternal recumbency, 35

Sternotomy, median, 90

Stress, 2

Stress leukogram, 8

Subcutaneous injection, 77

Sucralfate, 117

Suffering, 2

Surgical pain, 7

Sympatholytics, 25

T

Tachyphylaxis, prevention of, 10

Tepxalin, 24t

Thiopental
with castration, 85

with degloving injury, 99
with ear canal ablation, 102
for head trauma, 79
with hind limb amputation/
fracture, 97
with ovariohysterectomy, 83-84
with perianal fistula, 101

Thoracotomy, canine, 90-92

Tolfenamic acid, 24t

Topical anesthetic preparations,
local, 31-32

Torbutrol, 33t

Touhy needle
in epidural catheterization, 38-40
in intrapleural anesthesia, 63

Tourniquet, 58

Tramadol
dosages and indications for, 26t
with hind limb amputation/
fracture, 97
oral preparations of, 33t
for osteosarcoma-related pain, 117

Tranquilizers
for chronic pain, 109
in initial pain management, 77

Transcutaneous acupoint electrical
stimulation (TAES), 73

Transcutaneous electrical nerve
stimulation (TENS), 73

Transdermal opioid delivery
complications and
contraindications for, 70
drugs and dosages in, 70
materials needed for, 70
technical skills for, 70
technique in, 68-70

Transduction, 6

Transmission, 6

Trauma
head, 78-79
initial pain management for,
76-77

Tricyclic antidepressants
for chronic pain, 109, 111
dosages and indications for, 26t
with intervertebral disc
disease, 93

Tuberculin syringe, 52

U

V

W

X

Notes

Notes

Notes

Notes

Notes

Notes

Recommended Readings

Boothe, Dawn M. *Compounding: Astounding or Confounding? Proceedings, North American Veterinary Conference.* Volume 18, Number 2, 847-849, 2004.

Buback, Janice L, Boothe, Harry W, Carroll, Gwendolyn L, Green, Ronald W. Comparison of three methods for relief of pain after ear canal ablation. *Veterinary Surgery.* Volume 25: 380-385, 1996.

Carpenter, Rachael E, Wilson, Deborah V, Evans, Tom A. Evaluation of intraperitoneal and incisional lidocaine or bupivacaine for analgesia following ovariohysterectomy in the dog. *Veterinary Anesthesia and Analgesia,* Volume 31: 46-52, 2004.

Carrol, Gwendolyn L. *Small Animal Pain Management.* Lakewood, CO, AAHA Press, 1998

Craig, A D. Interoception: the sense of the physiological condition of the body. *Current Opinions in Neurobiology* Volume 13:500-505, 2003.

Dunning, Dianne, and Houlton, John. Perioperative patient management. *AO Principals of Fracture Management in Small Animals* (In Press).

Fiorucci, Stefano, Distrutti, Eleonora, Menezes De Lima, Octavio, et al. Relative contribution of acetylated cyclo-oxygenase (COX -2) and 5- lipoxygenase(LOX) in regulating gastric mucosal integrity and adaptation to aspirin. *FASEB Journal.* Volume 17: 1171-1173. 2003.

Flecknell, Paul and Waterman-Pearson, A. *Pain Management in Animals.* W.B. Saunders, London, 2000.

Gaynor, James and Muir, William W. *Handbook of Veterinary Pain Management.* Mosby, St. Louis, IL, 2002.

Greene, SA. Ed. *Veterinary Anesthesia and Pain Management Secrets.* Hanley and Belfus Inc. Philadelphia, 2002.

Hansen, Bernie. Analgesic Therapy in Critically Ill Patients. In *Predictable Pain Management.* United States, Veterinary Learning Systems, 1996

Hansen, Bernie. Management of Postoperative Pain in Dogs and Cats. In *Predictable Pain Management.* United States, Veterinary Learning Systems, 1996.

Hardie, Elizabeth M. Chronic Pain. In *Predictable Pain Management.* United States, Veterinary Learning Systems, 1996

Hardie, Elizabeth M. Management of Acute Pain. In *New Advances in Control of Pain and Inflammation.* United States, Veterinary Learning Systems, 1998.

Johnston, Spencer A. Physiology, Mechanisms, and Identification of Pain. In *Predictable Pain Management.* United States, Veterinary Learning Systems, 1996.

McMillan, Frank D. A World of Hurts – is Pain Special? JAVMA Volume 223(2):183-186, 2003.

Muir, William W, and Birchard, Stephen J. *Questions and Answers on Analgesia, Anesthesia, and Sedation.* United States, Veterinary Learning Systems, 1997.

Muir, William W, and Weise, Ashley J. Effect of Morphine, lidocaine, ketamine and morphine-lidocaine-ketamine drug combination on minimum alveolar concentration in dogs anesthetized with isoflurane. AJVR Volume 64(9):1155-1160, 2003.

Paddleford, Robert R. Analgesia and Pain Management. In *Manual of Small Animal Anesthesia.* 2nd Edition. Philadelphia, W.B. Saunders Company, 1999.

Papich, Mark G, and Hardie, Elizabeth M. Management of Chronic Pain. In *New Advances in Control of Pain and Inflammation.* United States, Veterinary Learning Systems, 1998.

Tomlinson, Julia and Blikslager, Anthony. Role of nonsteroidal anti-inflammatory drugs in gastrointestinal tract injury and repair. JAVMA, Volume 222(7):946-951. 2003.

Tranquilli, William, Faggella, Alicia, Hellyer, Peter, Quandt, Jane and Weale, John. A Roundtable Discussion; Rethinking Your Approach to Sedation, Anesthesia, and Analgesia. In *Veterinary Medicine,* Volume 92, Number 11. Lenexa, KS, 1997.

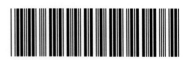